The
Canyon Ranch Guide
to Weight Loss

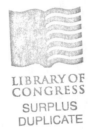

The Canyon Ranch® Guide to Weight Loss

A Scientifically Based Approach to Achieving and Maintaining Your Ideal Weight

Stephen C. Brewer, MD, ABFM
Medical Director of Canyon Ranch

With a Foreword by Jeff Kuster,
CEO of Canyon Ranch

Recipes by Stephanie Miezin, MS, RD, CSSD
Canyon Ranch Director of Nutrition

SelectBooks, Inc.
New York

This edition published by SelectBooks, Inc.
For information address SelectBooks, Inc., New York, New York.

First Edition

ISBN 978-1-59079-552-1

Library of Congress Cataloging-in-Publication Data

Names: Brewer, Stephen C., 1952- author. | Kuster, Jeff, author of
  foreword. | Miezin, Stephanie, contributor.
Title: The Canyon Ranch weight loss program : an integrated, sustainable
  plan to lose weight and feel great / Stephen C. Brewer, MD, ABFM,
  Medical Director of Canyon Ranch ; with a foreword by Jeff Kuster, CEO
  of Canyon Ranch ; recipes by Stephanie Miezin, MS, RD, Canyon Ranch
  Director of Nutrition.
Description: First edition. | New York : SelectBooks, [2023] | Includes
  bibliographical references and index. | Summary: "Medical director of
  Canyon Ranch introduces a weight-loss program designed to help many
  people, especially those feeling destined to fail at permanently
  dropping unwanted pounds. Exploring various topics about weight and
  general health, he provides recipes and advises moderate changes in diet
  and exercise to become healthier-and in the process lose weight and keep
  it off"-- Provided by publisher.
Identifiers: LCCN 2022028297 (print) | LCCN 2022028298 (ebook) | ISBN
  9781590795521 (hardcover) | ISBN 9781590795538 (ebook)
Subjects: LCSH: Reducing diets--Popular works.
Classification: LCC RM222.2 .B758 2023 (print) | LCC RM222.2 (ebook) |
  DDC 613.2/5--dc23/eng/20220824
LC record available at https://lccn.loc.gov/2022028297
LC ebook record available at https://lccn.loc.gov/2022028298

Book design by Janice Benight

Manufactured in the United States of America
10 9 8 7 6 5 4 3 2 1

I would like to dedicate this book to all my patients that I have counseled over the years who have struggled with their weight. Their strength and courage to improve their health by making healthy lifestyle changes has been truly inspirational to my staff and me.

Contents

Foreword *Jeff Kuster, CEO of Canyon Ranch®*

Live younger, longer. It is hard to disagree with that goal. This is Dr. Stephen Brewer's ultimate desire for you, and this book will be your guide. Along the way, you will discover and come to understand much about weight loss. As you will see, shedding some pounds is a good objective. But even better is learning how to do this in a healthy and sustainable way that is positive and enjoyable rather than grudging and restrictive.

With rare exceptions, the average life expectancy world-wide has been increasing constantly as long as records have been kept. In my life alone, since the 1960s, it has increased nearly ten years in the United States. Simply put—we are living longer. But how can we best savor those years in good health: fit, vital and engaged? There are so many competing voices in "the wellness industry" that it is easy to be confused or overwhelmed.

Dr. Brewer has long understood that we all need practical guidance that is factual, insightful, and simple. That is the purpose of this book. You might just need a nudge to get back on track, or you could be seeking details and a deeper understanding of the impact of diet and lifestyle on your health and weight. No matter where you are in your wellness journey, there is a lot to learn here.

I first met Dr. Brewer when I came to Canyon Ranch as a guest a few years ago. I was typical of many first timers. I was feeling that my life could be better. I started thinking that I wanted to lose weight and get healthier. My wife was already a Canyon Ranch fan having stayed several years previously. I remember thinking that I would take a few classes, get to the gym a bit, and just take a break. However, I soon found myself in Dr. Brewer's office, and my expectations changed—dramatically.

Weight loss starts with information, understanding and, perhaps most importantly, with empathy. It is hard to be open to advice and guidance when you feel like just a 10-minute blip in the day of a busy, impersonal medico. As with all of the experts at Canyon Ranch, Dr. Brewer saw me as a person, not a patient. Beyond his encyclopedic knowledge, he is a compassionate and caring partner. You know from the start that he is on your side, and you want to hear what he has to say.

And you would be hard pressed to find someone who has more authority and experience on the topic of healthy weight loss and sustainable health habits. Dr. Brewer has over forty years of medical practice and specializes in integrated medicine, the healing-oriented medicine that takes into account the whole person, including all aspects of lifestyle. It emphasizes the therapeutic relationship between practitioner and patient, is informed by evidence, and makes use of all appropriate therapies. For almost twenty years, he has served as the Medical Director at Canyon Ranch, and he has helped thousands of people understand how their bodies work, how to achieve their weight and fitness goals, and how to establish and maintain healthy habits. He has seen wellness fads come and go, but his approach has stood the test of time.

Dr. Brewer's thesis is straightforward. Sustainable, healthy weight loss is not based on any quick fixes. Neither does it require dramatic, life-altering behavioral change. His approach is that small changes, better choices, and consistent behavior can make an enormous difference for you over time. The benefits begin immediately, and they accrue steadily. At the same time, you will drop pounds and trim your waistline. Your commitment, however, must be holistic and systemic. Your medical condition, diet, nutrition, fitness, and emotional state all need to be addressed and engaged. Spoiler alert: Dr. Brewer's technique is indistinguishable from that of Canyon Ranch as a whole. All of the elements of your being—mind, body, and spirit—play a part, and each benefit from the other's improvements.

On that first day, I left Dr. Brewer's office to start a week-long immersion in learning, practicing, and living a better way of life. Empowered by Dr. Brewer's advice, I ate moderate portions of delicious, healthful, and natural food. I prioritized sleep. I learned not just when to exercise, but how to exercise. I added mindfulness and a sense of deeper purpose to my day. I quickly started to feel energized and optimistic. Then I had an "aha" moment. I realized that living a well way of life was not something I had to do; it was something I wanted to do. I realized the behaviors required were not only simple but enjoyable. With Dr. Brewer on my team to connect the dots and arm me with the tools I needed, I was ready and eager to return home inspired.

By picking up this book, you now have Dr. Brewer on your personal team to give you straight talk and realistic guidance. For many, this will be the first time that you have encountered this information presented in such a clear and concise manner. You will find new insights into optimizing your daily routine by gaining a better understanding of your body. With this knowledge and your own conviction, you will have the tools and courage to follow through and achieve your goals.

As a reward for your efforts, you are also going to find wonderful recipes in this book that will put to rest any concerns you may have that healthful, sensible food can be indulgent and satisfying. I often hear from guests at Canyon Ranch that they want to come home with special tips and tricks to give them an extra edge to stay engaged in their journey. It may seem counter-intuitive, but in your quest for weight loss and health, your ally will be these simply delicious and flavorful gourmet dishes.

Ultimately, transformation is a profound and personal thing. While it can be difficult for adults to change, you are about to discover that it is not only possible but easily attainable. Dr. Brewer has laid out the blueprint for you to follow. Soon you will be a master of the elements that impact weight and health. You are moments away from the wisdom and inspiration to live your well way of life.

—JEFF KUSTER, CEO OF CANYON RANCH

Acknowledgments

I would like to express my gratitude to Canyon Ranch for giving me the opportunity to work at one of the top wellness facilities in the world. I want to thank John Goff, the owner of Canyon Ranch, and Jeff Kuster, the CEO of Canyon Ranch, for supporting me at Canyon Ranch following the transition of ownership. They allowed me to grow and helped me to continue to develop our phenomenal integrative medical department. And I want to recognize Dustin Nabhan, DC, PhD., the VP of Health and Performance, and thank him for having confidence in me to advance my role as the Medical Director of Canyon Ranch.

I owe a very special thank-you to nutritionist Stephanie Miezin, MS, RD, CSSD, Director of Nutrition for Canyon Ranch®, for developing the recipes that were written for this book. Many an hour was put into not only writing these recipes but making sure they complemented what was discussed in the book. I would like to thank my partner, Diane Downing, MD, who is always there to discuss with me some of my more difficult cases. I want to extend gratitude to the rest of the Canyon Ranch Directors of Health and Performance that include Mike Siemens, MS, Director of Sports Science; Co-Directors of Mind and Spirit, Amy Hawthorne, MS, and Teresa Cowan Jones, MDiv; and Carlos Jimenez, DPT, SCS, CSCS, Canyon Ranch Director of Sports Medicine; for giving me great insights over the years about how to address weight loss from their specific areas of expertise.

I would like to thank Anna Kreutz, the Administrative Director of Health and Performance of Canyon Ranch®, for her unwavering help and support. And I want to extend my acknowledgment to all the rest

And I want to extend my acknowledgment to all the rest of the nurses, medical assistants, medical schedulers, and administrative assistants for helping me maneuver through my daily workdays.

I would like to thank my editor Nancy Sugihara for all her time and effort in editing this book to make it more readable and enjoyable. I want to thank my publisher, Kenzi Sugihara and SelectBooks Marketing Director Kenichi Sugihara , for having the faith in me to once again publish another book. This is now my third book that has been published by SelectBooks. I want to thank my book agent Bill Gladstone who seamlessly connected all the business dots to help put this project in motion.

Finally, as with all my books, I wish to acknowledge the support I have received from my daughter, Elizabeth Brewer, B.S., who is a wellness instructor for one of the top corporations in Silicon Valley and is back in school furthering her education to earn her doctorate in clinical psychology.

And last but not least, I want to express my appreciation to my sister, Deborah Brewer, RN., who has always been there for all kinds of support, including her medical expertise and her personal encouragement, for my whole life.

Basics of Weight Loss

Introduction

If you are looking for a quick and easy way to lose weight, this may not be the book for you. Many books written about weight loss give people hope that they can lose a boatload of weight in a relatively short period of time. This isn't one of them. It's a book that directs you to better health habits, and in the process of improving your health and lifestyle you will lose weight.

This is not a personal success story about how I was able to lose 100 pounds by some secret formula. This is a book based on my 40 years of helping patients lose weight. During the first half of my career I was able to help patients lose weight by improving their lifestyles. However, it wasn't until I became Medical Director of Canyon Ranch, nearly 20 years ago that I was able to understand how a more comprehensive interdisciplinary approach was by far the most successful way to lose weight and maintain the weight loss. Our program is not based on any of the latest fads but is grounded in solid evidence-based medicine. This approach not only helps a person lose weight but, most importantly, helps an individual to reach an overall healthier state.

Being overweight has been as much a societal issue as a health issue. Society seems solely focused on the number of pounds a person has gained or lost, mainly in terms of how this improves their appearance. How many times have you seen an article in the tabloids about a movie star losing a certain number of pounds by committing to some trendy new Hollywood diet? It's rare to read about famous people changing their lives to become healthier. I am not saying that

3

it's unimportant to lose those extra pounds. There is no question that being overweight increases a person's risk for chronic disease. As a physician, my biggest worry about obesity is not the cosmetic concerns that most people are anxious about, but all the medical complications and diseases that can result from being overweight. A few of the illnesses we hope to prevent by losing weight are diabetes, cardiovascular disease, cancer, fatty liver disease, and even dementia.

However, the number of pounds we lose is only one part of the equation in enhancing our overall health. The best approach is to find a program that will maximize a person metabolically, physically, and emotionally. In the process of reaching an optimal state of health, a person will be able to lose and be successful in keeping those extra pounds off. This enhanced healthy state gives a person a better chance to increase their longevity by decreasing their risk for developing a chronic disease and improve their overall quality of life.

By the time I see a patient at Canyon Ranch for weight loss, they have already tried many ways to lose weight. They have likely tried diets like the Keto diet or the blood type diet or experimented with intermittent fasting. They may have attempted to lose weight by exhausting themselves with some strenuous new exercise program. Committing to these often quick-fix plans may result in rapid weight loss, but there is no guarantee that they can keep those pounds off or, what's more significant, if they are healthier as a result. This book is about improving your health and keeping your extra pounds off for the long haul.

Over the years I have seen many patients who have tried to lose weight by partaking in various extreme dieting or exercise programs. Unfortunately, there can be major flaws with this approach. First of all, they rarely maintain these strict diets and exacting exercise programs. The far majority don't want to continue to starve themselves or spend endless hours pushing their limits. My patients may have lost weight and sometimes very rapidly, but few people can follow such difficult routines for long. We know life should be about living well—not about giving up our favorite foods and feeling exhausted every day. Unfortunately, because most people can't keep up with their rigorous programs, these once victorious people often gain back much of the weight they had worked so hard to drop. In some cases they may gain back more pounds than what they lost in the first place.

As I have been saying, losing weight is a good goal but is not always enough to improve our health. An example of this is my patient Jane, who was excited about her success. Over a relatively short period of 6 months she had lost 30 pounds. When she came to see me, she brought a copy of her recent blood work and a copy of her blood work taken before losing the weight. I took one look at her blood tests and immediately asked if her secret formula to weight loss was the "Keto diet." She was a little surprised and caught off guard by my question. Her answer was yes, and she was curious about how I knew she was on that particular diet. The reason I surmised that she had been on a Keto diet was the fact that her cholesterol levels had significantly increased from her previous test results before she started the diet. Many people on a Keto-like diet eat a lot of meat and fat and avoid carbs. By eating fewer carbs they are able to lose weight. But with all the meat and fat they consume on this diet, it's not shocking that many who participate in this particular weight loss program end up with high cholesterol levels. Jane had achieved her goal to lose weight but had accomplished it in such an unhealthy way that she was now at a higher risk for cardiovascular disease. This was decidedly not a good way to lose weight.

When Covid-19 hit in the spring of 2020, it would be the first time in its 40 years of existence that Canyon Ranch® would be shut down for a finite period of time. This meant it would be the first time in all my years of practicing medicine that I would not be seeing patients.

With this hiatus in my practice I was presented with the rare opportunity of having time on my hands to start writing again. To begin a new manuscript for a book, I needed only to determine the main subject. The interesting and fun aspect of being an integrative family physician is that I never know what type of health issue will be presented to me. It could be anything from discussing ways to decrease a person's risk of developing diabetes to educating a patient about their atrial fibrillation or helping a patient deal with chronic headaches.

While my library of topics I could write about seemed endless, I decided I wanted to pick a topic that would be applicable to a large subset of the population. If I addressed it effectively, this could have a major impact on improving their lives. I have written and lectured on many topics of special interest to me, such as fibromyalgia, with its probable root cause appearing to be a complex medical syndrome called Central Sensitization.

Other topics I have frequently written and lectured about are related to men's and women's health issues. I wrote *The Canyon Ranch Guide to Men's Health* because I wanted men to care about their health and understand themselves better. My most recent book, *What Happened to Moderation?*, was based on my personal philosophy of how I approach health in general. I feel that each of us should address our health from a position of moderation. In other words, people don't have to run marathons to improve their health and fitness. When deciding the theme of my next book, I looked back on all of the medical issues I have witnessed in my practice. The one overriding health issue that kept resurfacing in my mind was weight gain and obesity. This medical problem has afflicted untold number of individuals of both sexes. It is a source of many disease states and complicates other health issues that may already exist.

The problem of weight gain also worsened over the past few years when it became one of the far-reaching effects of the pandemic. We immediately think of the direct consequences of just trying to survive Covid-19 when someone had the misfortune to be afflicted by it. This was especially problematic if the disease was contracted early on when we had few methods to combat the virus.

However, we suffered many other indirect consequences. In our attempts to prevent contagion and spreading of Covid-19, most of us were forced into some type of isolation from the general public. Initially, many of us who were privileged to be comfortable at home decided to work on self-improvement. Among other ambitions, we would use this "home time" to improve our health. But sadly, even though we had more time to exercise and improve our diets, many of us exercised less and ate more. When we prepared our meals, we often ate high-caloric comfort food instead of healthy nutritious food. The natural consequence of this unhealthy behavior was weight gain.

The rise in obesity prior to the pandemic was already a public health issue in the United States. For instance, in all the states and territories of the USA, well over 20% of adults are classified as being obese. Only the state of Colorado and the District of Columbia have the rate of obesity between 20 and 25%. All the rest of the states and territories are greater than 25%. The Midwest at 33.9% and the South at 33.3% had the highest prevalence of obesity, followed by the Northeast at 29.0% and the West at 27.4%.[1] This rise in obesity is shocking. If the numbers of patients I have seen struggling with excess weight since the beginning of the pandemic are an indication of how the rest of the country is doing, the amount of obesity in the future is going to be staggering.

I feel it's very important to point out that we should not be hung up on trying to attain some magical number for our weight. We can spend too much time and energy attempting to achieve our goal of what we perceive as a perfect weight when being healthier is what our true end point should be. Yes, if one is overweight, losing weight is important. But it is not usually the one answer to becoming healthier. I had one patient that followed to the "T" everything I suggested to improve her health. She ate wonderful healthy meals, exercised daily, slept well, and learned to de-stress.

Metabolically, she was doing wonderfully. All her blood sugars showed no glucose spikes after eating (I talk in chapter 3 about the potential negative consequences that may occur with blood glucose spikes), and all her other metabolic markers were right in the normal range. Despite this, she remained ten pounds heavier than what she wanted to be. During her visits to me I tried to encourage her by explaining how all her numbers were better than they had ever been. But she remained very frustrated.

One day I told her that based on all the excellent results of her blood work, if she continued to follow her prescribed exercise program, eating the recommended healthy meals, and in general practicing a healthy lifestyle, her future seemed very bright, indeed. I went on at some length to explain that her risk of getting a chronic disease was low, and the odds of her living well into her 90s was highly probable. After quietly listening to this report, it finally sank in. She looked at me straight in my eyes, gave me a wry smile, and admitted that she could probably stand to live with those extra ten pounds.

Canyon Ranch has been helping individuals lose weight for over forty years. Their secret "juice" is not rocket science. It is simply removing individuals from their unhealthy home and workspace and placing them in a wonderfully, healthy, structured place for a planned period of time. It's amazing how quickly the human body and mind can respond and flourish when in the right environment. The key is having what we call a "healthy structure." If we start to lose this daily structure, we may suddenly go ahead and have that extra helping of potatoes or "forget" about getting up early in the morning to exercise. To be successful in weight loss, one needs to maintain a structure. And it must be a healthy structure because, just like building a house, no matter how attractive it may look on the outside (like the body after weight loss), if the foundation is poorly built (if the body does not also become healthier as a result), the whole house will eventually cave in.

The importance of a healthy structure was pointed out to me years ago when I was at a conference at Duke University, and the person lecturing was my mentor, Dr. Andrew Weil. During the question and answer period of his talk, someone in the audience asked Dr. Weil what he thought of the diet named the "Blood Type Diet." Dr. Weil immediately said he thought it was a stupid diet but stated that it appeared to work in helping people lose weight. When everyone seemed puzzled by his answer, he explained himself. He told us that to his knowledge the blood-type diet had no real scientific basis, and that's why he felt it was stupid. He stated that each one of the blood type diets written were basically healthy, and if a person stuck to their blood type diet and didn't waver from it (for example: not having ice cream at bedtime because that's not part of your blood-type diet) they often lost weight because of the diet's healthy structure.

One last thing I want to mention in this introduction is the nature versus. nurture aspect of weight loss. If your parents are overweight, are you doomed to also be overweight? Most of this book is a discussion about the nurture aspects of weight loss, but we must acknowledge that nature does play a role in how our bodies are shaped. The heritability of increased body fat compared to the average individual is estimated from studies of twins can be high, ranging from 40 to 70% with slightly lower values with twins who are raised apart compared to twins raised together.[2] Similarly, the body mass index of adopted children was closer to their biologic parents than their adopted parents.

Over 500 fat-related genetic loci that have been discovered. The *FTO* (fat mass and obesity-associated) gene on chromosome 16 is one

of the strongest genes associated with obesity.[3] What this means ultimately is that if there is obesity in your family and you are overweight,
your path to weight loss can be more arduous. It certainly doesn't
mean you can't lose weight; it simply means you will probably have to
work harder at it than most people. So if you have obesity in your family, the earlier you embark on a healthy lifestyle, the better your odds
are of attaining your goals. In addition, since we know that we pass
our genes onto our offspring, it is important to realize that if you are
overweight and you have children, there is an increased chance your
children can be overweight. With that in mind, the earlier you start
your children on the road to healthy eating and exercise, the easier it
will be for them to grow up with normal weight. There is more detail
about genetics and weight loss in chapter 12.

1

Medical Causes of Weight Gain

When we gain weight, we are quick to blame over-eating, lack of exercise, or those chocolate chip cookies that are sitting right in front us at the grocery store checkout line. It is true: These are some of the more common reasons a person gains weight, but we always need to make sure there is not some underlying medical reason for those added pounds that can be corrected. An example of a medical problem associated with weight gain is an underactive thyroid that might be corrected by taking medicine. Therefore, before you decide to exercise for several hours every day or determine you should just starve yourself for a couple of weeks, please try to rule out potentially correctable causes of weight gain.

The length of time it took to gain those extra pounds can often give us clues about the source of that weight gain. If your putting on weight occurred in a relatively short period of time (that can be loosely defined as less than six months), it's appropriate to look for an underlying medical condition as a potential cause. Here are some of the more common medical causes of weight gain:

1. Hypothyroid (underactive thyroid)

2. Depression

3. Medications

4. Sleep disturbances

5. Menopause

6. Cushing's disease

7. Polycystic Ovary disease

8. Fluid retention: from organ dysfunction such as heart failure, liver disease or kidney disease.

9. Certain medical treatments for diabetes

10. Steroid treatments

Let's look at these medical maladies a little closer.

Hypothyroidism

I cannot tell you how many overweight people have come to see me over my decades of practicing medicine because they were convinced their weight gain was due to an underactive thyroid. This was especially common if they knew a family member who had a thyroid hormone deficiency and were able to have a significant loss of weight after their low thyroid activity was thankfully corrected.

It's true that an under-acting thyroid can cause weight gain. The thyroid hormone is responsible for controlling a person's metabolism. If it is under-producing, a person's metabolism slows down. When that happens people do not burn up as many calories as they normally do, and low and behold, they gain weight.

Ninety-five percent of low thyroid conditions are diagnosed as primary hypothyroidism, which means that for whatever reason the thyroid gland that is situated in the anterior portion of the neck, is under-producing the thyroid hormone. The other rare 5% of cases are secondary and tertiary hypothyroidism. "Secondary" means the disease is in the pituitary gland and "tertiary" means the problem is in the area of the brain that is above the pituitary gland called the "hypothalamus." Because these conditions are rare, l will not go into detail about these diseases. One should consider that the source of the hypothyroidism is a secondary or tertiary cause rather than a primary hypothyroidism if the thyroid hormone (T4) is low, the pituitary hormone TSH (which stands for thyroid stimulating hormone) is also low,[4] and these findings in a person are accompanied by the following:

○ There is a known hypothalamic or pituitary disease.

○ A mass lesion is present in the pituitary.

○ Symptoms and signs of hypothyroidism are associated with other hormone deficiencies.

Potential Complications of Hypothyroidism

Mechanism	Symptoms
Slowing of metabolic processes	Fatigue and weakness Cold intolerance Dyspnea on exertion Weight gain Cognitive dysfunction Mental retardation (infantile onset) Constipation Growth failure
Accumulation of matrix substances	Dry skin Hoarseness Edema
Other	Decreased hearing Myalgia and paresthesia Depression Menorrhagia (changes in a woman's menstruation) Arthralgia (joint pain)

Otherwise the other 95% of hypothyroidisms are diagnosed when a person has a low T4 and the TSH is elevated (when the pituitary gland is working overtime to try to stimulate the thyroid gland to produce thyroid hormones). It is important to note that at the beginning of this disease process the TSH will often be elevated before the T4 drops. This is sometimes called "subclinical hypothyroidism." It is much better to recognize and treat the problem at this stage than allowing the disease to progress and result in a significant gain in weight.

The causes of primary hypothyroidism, are:

○ Chronic autoimmune thyroiditis, which is called Hashimotos thyroiditis.

○ Iatrogenic (physician-induced) thyroidectomy and radiation therapy

○ Iodine deficiency

○ Drugs (this is not a totally inclusive list) such as thion-amides, lithium, amiodarone, interferon, interleukin-2, and tyrosine kinase inhibitors.

○ Infiltrative diseases: fibrous thyroiditis, hemochromato-sis, sarcoidosis

○ Transient hypothyroidism: This can be seen when some-one undergoes a serious stressful event such as a life-threatening illness that causes the thyroid to under function for a finite time.

○ Thyroiditis: painless, subacute, and often post-partum

○ Congenital thyroid agenesis, dysgenesis, or defects in hormone synthesis

If you are being analyzed about the possibility of a thyroid condition, these causes should be discussed with your doctor to help make a diagnosis. As mentioned earlier, there are two simple blood tests that can be performed to determine if a person has low-hormone producing thyroid disease. These tests are a TSH and T4. They will pick up low thyroid activity in the far majority of cases.

What we often do at Canyon Ranch is obtain additional thyroid blood tests. They are a T3 and thyroid antibodies. T4 converts to T3 and thyroid antibodies will be elevated if there is an autoimmune disease such as Hashimotos thyroiditis. These additional tests can occasionally help in understanding and managing a person's thyroid condition.

The symptoms of hypothyroid are not just weight gain. They can be quite varied and often depend on the extent of the hypothyroidism as shown in the list on page 13.[5]

Depression and Other Serious Mental Illnesses

Serious mental illnesses (SMI), including schizophrenia, bipolar disorder (BD), and major depressive disorder (MDD), have a two to three times higher mortality rate than the general population and ten to twenty years reduced life expectancy that appears to be widening. The majority of deaths in persons with SMI are caused by physical diseases that are predominantly cardiovascular diseases (CVDs).[6] Genetic and non-medical factors, including unhealthy lifestyles and disparities in health care, contribute to this increased prevalence. Another significant cause of this increased mortality is related to the weight gain that can be associated with abnormal eating behaviors and the medications used to treat their mental illness. Medications that cause weight gain are discussed in the next section.

Depression often results in higher measures of emotional eating, and this predicts a greater increase in BMI (body mass index).[7] Disordered eating is common in individuals suffering from emotional disorders, especially those suffering from depression. Appetite and weight may decrease or increase during states of depression and premenstrual disorders. Some patients have to force themselves to eat, whereas others eat more and may crave specific foods (for example: junk food and carbohydrates). Unfortunately, individuals that are already overweight and then suffer a major depressive episode are five times more likely to overeat compared to people who start off with a normal weight and then become depressed.[8]

Some simple advice is this: If you find that a black cloud of depression is slipping into your life, please don't wait till the sky is pouring cats and dogs. Talk to your doctor or therapist about your feelings of sadness and depression before disordered eating overwhelms you and the pounds come rolling in. More of the emotional aspect of weight gain is discussed in chapter 9.

Pharmaceuticals are one of the common treatments for depression. There is a potential for side effects with any medication. Unfortunately, as effective as many of drugs are for the treatment of depression and other mental illnesses, one of their common side effects is weight gain.

Medications and Weight Gain

One of the first questions I ask a patient with newly onset weight gain is if they had recently been placed on a new medication. There are various mechanisms involved in drug-induced weight gain. Examples are fluid retention and increased appetite. The following are some of the more common medications that can result in weight gain

Antidepressant and Antipsychotic Medications

I have noticed over the years that a significant number of my patients with depression have struggled with their weight. (Depression-induced weight gain will be discussed in detail in chapter 9.) What puzzled me was that when a psychiatrist or I treated my patients with antidepressants, they often seemed to gain even more weight. It didn't take long for me to surmise that somehow many of these antidepressants were a probable source for their weight gain. The pharmaceutical companies tried to deny this, but over time many scientific studies were produced that backed up what I was seeing clinically.[9]

There are several chemically distinct antidepressants. There are the older tricyclic antidepressants such as amitriptyline (brand name

Elavil), the SSRIs like fluoxetine (brand name Prozac), the combination drugs like venlafaxine (brand name Effexor) and mirtazapine (brand name Remeron), that are both noradrenergic and seratonergic, and there are drugs that increase dopamine such as bupropion (brand name Wellbutrin).

Tricyclic antidepressants are one of the oldest groups of antidepressants. These include such drugs as amitriptyline, doxepin and nortriptyline. All of these drugs can be associated with weight gain. They also have a lot of other side effects like dry mouth and drowsiness. These drugs are still occasionally used as antidepressants but are more commonly used to help people fall sleep or treat chronic pain syndromes.

The next major group of antidepressants to come along was the Selective Serotonin Reuptake Inhibitors (SSRIs). Prozac was the original drug in this group. They work by increasing the neurotransmitter called serotonin. When they were first introduced, they were touted as being the new miracle treatment for depression. They had a lot of advantages over the tricyclics. They had fewer side effects and it was much easier to regulate their dosages. In this class of medications there are certain ones that are more likely to cause weight gain than others. The two most notable for weight gain are paroxetine and sertraline.[10]

In the first line antidepressants that are more weight neutral and less likely to cause weight gain are duloxetine (brand name Cymbalta), a combination drug, bupropion (brand name Wellbutrin) that increases dopamine, and fluoxetine (brand name Prozac), a SSRI. I will often direct patients to consider these drugs when weight is an issue and urge them to discuss it with their therapist to see if it is possible to switch to these more weight-neutral antidepressants.

When individuals have severe forms of depression, and the first line of antidepressants are only partially effective, psychiatrists may add an antipsychotic medication to go along with their antidepressant medication. These medications can be life changing for people with clinical severe depression. Antipsychotics are also used for other major mental illnesses such as schizophrenia-spectrum disorders and bipolar disorder. Unfortunately these drugs are also associated with weight gain. The gain in weight is greatest with the second-generation antipsychotic agents clozapine and olanzapine, as compared to first generation agents iloperidone, quetiapine, risperidone, paliperidone, sertindole, and zotepine, which confer an intermediate risk of weight gain. Other antipsychotics that are associated with a small increase in body weight are amisulpride, aripiprazole, asenapine, lurasidone and ziprasidone.[11]

The question that arises is: Why do taking these medications cause you to gain weight? There is some dispute about this, but studies have shown that both the antidepressants and the antipsychotics are associated with an increase in a person's appetite and an increase in food intake as well as a delayed satiety signaling. (In other words you don't sense that your stomach is full until you have already eaten another helping of potatoes!). This is a result of stimulating the serotonin (5-HT2C) and histamine (H1) receptors.[12] With antipsychotics there may be an additional effect by adversely affecting insulin sensitivity and secretion.[13] Finally there is evidence that certain antipsychotics adversely affect the microbiome in such a way that it can cause weight gain.[14]

Cortisone and other Steroids

Cortisone has long been known to cause weight gain. It is commonly used for various disease states in which inflammation is the major culprit. This is seen in diseases like rheumatoid arthritis and other autoimmune diseases. It is used for various lung conditions such as asthma and different types of allergic reactions. In addition it is used for many skin maladies. Cortisone is an excellent medication and has been lifesaving for many conditions. However, when it is used for a prolonged period of time, it has a lot of potential side effects—one of which is weight gain. There are various reasons for this. Cortisones increase a person's appetite and causes the body to retain fluid. It also mobilizes sugars and fats and can affect insulin secretion. All of these can lead to gaining weight.

It is important to note that cortisone medications cannot be stopped cold turkey. Sudden cessation of this drug, especially if it has been at a high dose for a long time can cause severe medical issues. You could have a life-threatening reaction of low blood pressure. If you and your physician decide you should discontinue this drug, it must slowly be weaned down under the watchful eye of your health care provider.

Antihistamines

Antihistamines are commonly used drugs by the general public. They are effective in the treatment of allergies and are used broadly because they are easily obtained over the counter without a prescription. Because of their widespread use, most people do not know that antihistamines have been associated with weight gain. This was found to be true with certirizine (Zyrtec) , fexofenadine (Allegra) and deslortatadine (Clarinex). [15] They don't necessarily increase a person's appetite but work by blocking a person's sensation of feeling full.

Anti-seizure Medications

Medications used to prevent seizures are another potential source of weight gain. The seizure meds most likely to cause weight gain are Carbamazepine, gabapentin, valproate.[16] It is important to know that these medications, in additions to being used to prevent seizures, are being used more and more for chronic pain syndromes and emotional illnesses. Some of the more weight neutral anti-seizure meds are topiramate and lamotrigine.

Beta-Blockers

These medications slow the heart rate down, which helps treat high blood pressure and heart rhythm disturbances. With a slower heart rate an individual is often fatigued, and they have less of desire to be active. Even if they want to exercise, they have a difficult time performing high intensity workouts because of the governor effect of the medication. With these effects it is not surprising that in the *Journal of Gastroenterology* (May 2017) it showed that a person's metabolism is slowed with beta-blockers, which ultimately decreases the ability to burn calories.[17]

Diabetic Medications

There are several medications used to treat diabetes that can increase the risk of gaining weight. We all know that insulin is essential for life. Its job is to take glucose from the blood and place it into the cell to be utilized for energy. The problem with insulin is if there is excess it can result in storing fat. When I first started practicing medicine in the early 1980s, we were learning the importance of getting a person's blood sugars under tight control to avoid the potential complications associated with diabetes. Some of those complications are diabetic retinopathy (eye disease), diabetic neuropathy (nerve injury) and diabetic nephropathy (kidney damage). The feeling at the time was to start using insulin early in the treatment rather than focusing on lifestyle changes to control blood sugars. I must point out here that I am now discussing Type II diabetes, which is about insulin resistance and the inability of insulin to work as well rather than the underproduction or lack of production of insulin that is seen in Type I diabetes. I followed this preferred therapy and placed many of my patients on insulin relatively early in the course of their disease. When these patients returned to see me in follow-up, I began to notice an unfortunate trend. Even though their blood sugars were under better control, many were gaining weight. This was quite discouraging because the majority of these patients were overweight to begin with. I would readjust their insulin, mostly by increasing their dose and have them return to my clinic in two to four weeks. The same thing would happen. They would have okay blood sugar control but progressive weight gain. It all started when I placed these individuals on insulin early in the course of their disease rather than directing them to change their lifestyles and lose weight.

I must say right now that if you are already taking insulin, DO NOT STOP your insulin because of what you just read here. That could have serious consequences. Many diabetics need to be on insulin. What I am addressing here is the possibility of decreasing or even preventing the use of insulin in the first place. By healthy eating, regular exercising, improving sleep habits, learning to de-stress, you might avoid the need to start taking insulin and can often prevent weight gain.

Our bodies produce insulin in the pancreas. For the treatment of diabetes there are medications that can cause the body to make more insulin and were the original non-insulin drugs used to treat Type II diabetes. These early agents to increase pancreatic secretion of insulin are called sulfonylureas, and they can successfully reduce a person's blood sugar levels, Sulfonylureas include gliclazide (Diamicron) and glibenclamide (Glynase). But unfortunately they also commonly cause weight gain, as noted in a study published in the Archives of Medical Science in 2015.[18]

Other medications used in treatment of diabetes are the following:

  ○ *Metformin* is another oral diabetic medication that is not a sulfonylurea. It is usually my first line medication treatment for those diabetics that are unable to get their blood sugars under control despite making excellent lifestyle changes. It appears to be weight neutral. It works by decreasing glucose production from the liver and by doing so actually decreases the need for insulin. When this happens a person's insulin levels are often lowered. This is an old drug but still a very good drug. Metformin has gotten a bad rap because some individuals have gastrointestinal symptoms with it. To prevent these symptoms this drug should be taken in the middle of the meal and not on an empty stomach. If you are a person who quit taking it in the past because it upset your stomach, I recommend trying it again by taking it in the middle of your meal and see what happens.

Three newer groups of diabetes medications are called GLP-1 (Glucagon-like peptide-1) agonists, SGLT2 (sodium-glucose cotransporter 2) inhibitors and DPP4 (Dipeptidyl peptidase 4) inhibitors. They, too, appear to be weight neutral and in some cases may cause weight loss.

○ *The GLP-1 agonist* works by slowing down the emptying of food through the stomach. It increases a person's feeling of fullness when eating by slowing down the transit time of food in the gut, decreases glucagon (glucagon's function is to release stored glucose) secretion, and increases insulin secretion. They have been found to have some benefit in weight loss. Much of this has to do with the feeling of fullness in the gut.

○ *SGLT2 inhibitors* reduce the reabsorption of glucose in the kidneys and therefore lowers a person's overall glucose level. The osmotic effect of glycosuria (glucose in the urine) causes a diuretic effect. With the resultant loss of excess fluid volume, there is often a benefit of weight loss.

○ *DPP-4 inhibitors* work by inhibiting the enzyme that breaks down GLP-1 and another hormone called glucose-dependent insulinotropic polypeptide (GIP). These drugs have been found to be more weight neutral

Menopausal Weight Gain

I feel I could write a lengthy book on this topic alone. Over my years of private practice, and now presently in my position as medical director at Canyon Ranch, I have been around a lot of menopausal women both personally and professionally. I have seen their frustration about suddenly being heavier and their dismay at the unwelcome reshaping of their bodies, including the redistribution of fat from the hips to the midline that occurs around the time of menopause. The startling scientific fact is that over 40 percent of women ages 45 to 60 are not just overweight but considered obese.[19]

So what's going on here? Let's look at the scientific facts about this time of life for women. Studies have shown that starting around two years before menopause, women's physical activity decreases and remains this way after they have gone through menopause.[20] There are various psychosocial reasons for this. This is often the sandwich phase in their lives when many women are taking care of parents on one end and on the other end are helping out demanding older children and young grandchildren. This is also a time when many women are trying to juggle the demands of a booming career. With so many things pulling at them from different directions, the thought of finding time to exercise five days a week is often not in the cards. So when this happens that old mathematical equation once again comes into play: energy consumption minus energy expenditure = weight gain or loss. When you don't burn up that consumed energy, the simple response is gaining a few or a lot of pounds.

Women barely have enough time to do any cardio exercises (running, fast walking, swimming, cycling, rowing, etc.), let alone have time for weight training. When we don't spend time pumping iron we lose muscle mass. This is a deadly sin because, as will be discuss more in the exercise chapter, we must maintain—or in some cases increase—our muscle mass to be able to burn up calories. Remember, our muscles are the calorie burning factories of the body, and the more muscles you have, the more calories you can burn.

The other obvious elephant in the room is the reduction of estrogen during this perimenopausal time. Sex hormones play an essential role in the regulation of appetite, eating behavior, and energy metabolism.[21] Estrogen appears to suppress a woman's appetite and the distribution of adipose tissue, a name for body fat. There is a direct effect of estrogen on the hypothalamus, which suppresses a women's appetite.[22] Estrogen also appears to increase the production of leptin. Leptin is a hormone produced in the body that is one of the body's strongest appetite suppressants. [23] Therefore, when estrogen levels decrease with perimenopause, leptin levels will also decrease. Another factor that increases a woman's appetite is that levels of the "hunger hormone," ghrelin, have been found to be significantly higher among perimenopausal women compared to premenopausal and postmenopausal women.[24]

With this increased appetite, studies have shown that women's intake of dietary protein, carbohydrate, and fiber is significantly higher three to four years before the onset of menopause. In addition to the increased appetite and increased food intake during this time, fat oxidation (the ability to break down fat) appears to also be affected by a women's hormonal changes. Fat oxidation was decreased by 32% in women who became postmenopausal.[25]

The metabolic effects of menopause on a women's body are:[26]

1. Increasing central obesity (that midline bulge) with changes in the fat tissue distribution from the hips to the belly.

2. Potential increase in insulin resistance. Insulin is not as effective, and therefore the body has to make more insulin

to transport glucose into the cells. As already stated, higher insulin levels cause more fat storage.

3. Changes in serum lipid concentrations (cholesterol levels), which seems to be associated with increasing weight.

4. There appears to be an association between menopause and hypertension.[27]

Another common problem with perimenopausal women is poor sleep, and lack of sleep is commonly associated with weight gain. There are two hormonal causes for not having a good night's sleep. One is a lack of estrogen. This causes hot flashes, and when this occurs at night, it can disrupt sleep. The second is progesterone. When ovulation stops or is infrequent, the production of progesterone is lowered because its production originates from the corpus luteum, which forms in the ovary after ovulation. This hormone is helpful for women to fall asleep and stay asleep. The effects of poor sleep will be discussed in the next section, but suffice it to say that not having enough sleep often makes us more hungry than usual the next day.

Because much of a women's weight gain is a result of female hormone depletion, hormone replacement therapy may be of some benefit. It can certainly help sleep and may decrease appetite and increase metabolic rate. It may also improve insulin sensitivity. This is a discussion that needs to be held between you and your doctor. If there is a strong family history of female cancer or a personal experience of cancer, the use of hormone replacement may not be a good recommendation.

Lack of Sleep and Weight Gain

The rise in obesity has coincided with a decline in the number of individuals who report regularly obtaining the recommended seven to nine hours of sleep. Many people are sleeping fewer than six hours a night. Insufficient sleep is a risk factor of weight gain and obesity. There are many causes of insufficient sleep. One area encompassing a lot of sleep problems is "disordered sleep." This includes such problems as sleep apnea (stopping breathing for more than ten seconds an episode), insomnia (not being able to fall asleep or stay asleep), shortened sleep time, restless leg syndrome, and as discussed in the previous section, disrupted sleep (such as having a nighttime of hot flashes common with menopause. The mechanisms associated with insufficient sleep and weight gain include; changes in satiety and hormones that alter food intake and EE (Energy expenditure). Insufficient sleep is associated with decreases in the satiety hormone leptin and increases in the hunger-stimulating hormone ghrelin. It has also been hypothesized that when chronic lack of sufficient sleep reduces EE (Energy expenditure), this leads to weight gain.[28] Basically, this makes sense, since who wants to exercise when they are tired?

An interesting study that specifically looked at sleep loss and weight gain showed that the total daily food intake, especially of carbohydrates, was greater during times of poor sleeping. That additional intake of food was usually seen in the evenings after dinner. The consuming of carbohydrates, protein, and fiber calories after dinner in that study was 42 percent higher during times of sleep loss. This study also pointed out that participants often ate smaller breakfasts in the morning after insufficient sleep. These food changes are a result of a person's delay in their circadian timing of eating that can occur with insufficient sleep.[29] The importance of eating breakfast and meal timing will be discussed later under the section of weight loss maintenance.

Increased food intake during periods of not sleeping well appears to be a physiological adaptation to provide the body with the energy needed to sustain extended wakefulness. However, when exposed to the modern weight-gaining environment of readily accessible food, those pounds start adding up because food intake is more than necessary to offset the energy cost of sleep loss. This weight gain can be exacerbated if physical exhaustion leads to a reduced physical activity in the work–home environment. Even with studies showing increased hunger with loss of sleep, it does not completely explain the amount of overeating that was observed in the scientific studies. For that reason the sleep scientific world feels there is something else happening, most likely in the brain, that can explain such excess overeating that is seen when we don't get enough sleep.[30]

So when should you suspect that you have a sleep disturbance you are not aware of? The first clue is how you feel when you get out of bed in the morning. Do you feel well rested or do you feel like you could go back to sleep for another couple hours? If you don't feel rested, you could have some form of sleep disturbance. The second clue is how you feel during the day. Are you often tired? Do you fall asleep easily during the day while watching TV or sitting as a passenger in a car? A third major clue can come from the person's bed partner who more often than not can tell you if you are not sleeping well. They may observe their partner having excessive leg or arm movement, which is called restless leg syndrome or having episodes of prolonged pauses in their breathing, called sleep apnea. These apneic episodes are often immediately followed by a gasping for air that may or may not wake that person up. If you have any of these clues, please discuss it with your doctor. Your physician will decide if any further studies should be done to determine if you have a true sleep disturbance that may be contributing to your weight gain.

Polycystic Ovary Syndrome (PCOS)

PCOS is the most common hormonal disorder in women of child-bearing age. It has an odd name since many women diagnosed with this syndrome do not have cysts on their ovaries. Some of the clues that a woman may have PCOS are: They are of childbearing age, have

problems with infertility, have symptoms of erratic menstrual periods, and have growth of facial hair. Finally it is not uncommon for
women who have this syndrome to be overweight.

There are two major features noted with this syndrome: One is
that women with PCOS are insulin resistant. As a result of this insulin resistance, the body has to make higher levels of insulin to get glucose into the cells. This higher level of insulin in itself can increase
fat storage. The second feature of PCOS is that these women often
produce an excess amount of the male hormone, testosterone. This
is a result of the direct effect of high insulin onto the ovaries and has
been shown to increase male hormone production.[31] This in turn can
cause signs of "male-pattern baldness" (a condition of increased loss
of hair on the scalp all too familiar to middle-aged men who experience a receding hairline and thinning of hair on the crown), and they
may develop significant acne. This elevated production of androgens
is also a major factor in reshaping a women's body from their normal
pear shape to a more male apple shape. Lifestyle changes that include
a more calorie-restrictive diet and stepped-up exercise program has
been shown to help decrease the excess amounts of insulin.

In addition to the lifestyle changes, the medication metformin
is commonly added to the therapeutic regime to treat this condition.
As discussed earlier in this chapter, metformin decreases the production of glucose from the liver. With less glucose around, the body
will make less insulin. With lower insulin levels there is less fat storage and less production of the male androgens from the ovaries. This
ultimately can help to facilitate weight loss and hopefully prevents the
male-pattern fat deposition commonly known as "belly fat."

Weight Gain from Organ Diseases

Weight gain can occur from fluid retention related to certain underlying diseases. This is a very serious problem that must be addressed. I
have had patients come to see me requesting a diet plan because they

had gained a significant amount of weight in a relatively short period of time. Rapid weight gain is often a red flag that something more is going on in the body than simply eating too many jelly donuts. It can be a sign that there is a serious underlying medical issue that can be the source of that weight gain. An example of this was my patient Mary. She came to see me because she had gained 40 pounds in 6 months. I noticed that she had significant swelling in her legs. When I squeezed them, they felt soft and mushy, and they left imprints of my fingers when I removed my hand. This is called pitting edema. I then checked her blood count, and it was 7. This meant she had severe anemia. It was about half the amount of red blood cells a person normally has. I admitted her immediately to the hospital and gave her a blood transfusion because of her life-threatening low blood count. I then consulted a gastroenterologist to perform an endoscopy and colonoscopy to look for a possible source of blood loss from an internal bleed such as an ulcer or a colon cancer.

No source of bleeding was found during her endoscopy. But what the gastroenterologist found shocked us both. In the first part of her small intestine, called the duodenum, the lining showed a very shiny surface area that appeared abnormal to the gastroenterologist. He took biopsies of the unusual looking tissue. Under the pathologist's microscopic they found a loss of the normal villi that line the duodenum. The villi are very small microscopic protrusions into the lumen of the duodenum. These villi exponentially increase the surface area of the duodenum. This allows the body to absorb the healthy nutrients ingested. The loss of surface area in the patient's gut severely compromised her ability to absorb the food and nutrients necessary for a healthy existence. It was literally starving her.

Protein and iron were among the many nutrients she was unable to absorb. Protein in the blood stream holds blood fluid through oncotic pressure in the blood vessels and keeps it from diffusing out into the tissues. When there isn't enough protein in the blood stream, fluid seeps out and causes swelling of ankles and legs. That was the source of Mary's leg swelling and weight gain. Her severe anemia was a result of not absorbing iron across the gut and therefore an inability to make red blood cells.

When I put this patient in the hospital, she was in critical condition. She was placed on very strong intravenous anti-inflammatory medication to heal the lining of her small intestine and rebuild the villi in her gut. Once the gut wall was healed, she was able to retain the protein she ingested. This helped keep her blood fluid in the blood stream and not in the tissues. To speed things along she was also given IV diuretics to remove the excess fluid.

The source of the women's illness was determined to be celiac disease. Individuals with this disease have an immunologic reaction to gluten that severely damages the intestinal wall and wipes out a significant amount of a person's villi when gluten is ingested. Gluten is a protein found in wheat, barley, and rye. This was in the early 1990s, and the medical field at that time felt that celiac was an extremely rare genetic disease that the general practitioner would probably never see. We now know the true incidence of celiac is about one person in 137 people. It should be noted that although many people think they have celiac illness, most do not have the true disease. They may have indigestion from eating gluten, but they do not have the true genetic disease that can cause all the problems this patient developed.

After my patient stopped all gluten and completed her course of anti-inflammatory medications, her gut lining began to heal. This permitted her gut to now absorb the nutrients, protein, and iron that she could not absorb in the past. By eliminating gluten in her diet, she was able to lead a healthy life and became 40 pounds lighter. If she had decided only to increase her exercise and decrease caloric intake to lose the weight, it could easily have threatened her life.

There are other diseases of our internal organs that can cause fluid retention. This can occur in people who have dysfunction of their heart, kidney, liver, or lungs. Of these particular organ diseases, heart disease is one of the more common causes of fluid retention and therefore increased weight gain. The heart, which works as a pump, accepts into its right-sided chamber the returned blood from the body that has used up its oxygen and contains carbon dioxide from cell metabolism. The heart then pumps the deoxygenated blood up to the lungs to exchange the carbon dioxide for fresh oxygen and then returns the blood to the left side of the heart. From its left side the heart pumps the oxygenated blood back out to the whole body to utilize the fresh oxygen for metabolism.

If the heart is not working well, it's like any other pump that isn't functioning properly. The fluid that is supposed to move forward slows down, and fluid starts to back up. There are multiple heart diseases that can cause the heart to dysfunction. One example is viral myocarditis. This has been seen in rare Covid-19 cases when the virus settles in the heart muscle and causes direct damage to the heart muscle itself. Having a heart attack certainly is another potential cause of having heart failure. Some individuals have what is called a silent heart attack in which their initial symptoms are fluid retention and weight gain. If your sump pump in the basement is not working during a rainstorm, your basement may fill up with water. Just like that malfunctioning sump pump, if your heart is not pumping well, just as your basement fills up with water, your legs and body start to hold fluid and swell. With this fluid retention a person's weight increases. The treatment is to get rid of that excess fluid with the use of diuretics and to find the root cause for the heart dysfunction and try to correct it, if possible.

People with liver and kidney diseases often experience weight gain. It is common to develop fluid retention in both of these states. of illness. I am not going to go into the complexities of these diseases and how fluid retention occurs, but what is important to know is that there are some very simple blood-screening tests can be used to rule in or out liver or kidney disease. These blood panels look for liver disease by measuring liver enzymes (AST, ALT, and GGT) and kidney disease by measuring the BUN and creatinine levels. If these blood tests are abnormal, you need to take a deeper dive into potential kidney or liver disease by working closely with your health-care provider.

In addition to the organ diseases we have discussed, there are other diseases of our organs that can potentially result in weight gain, such as chronic lung disease.

Loss of Muscle Mass from Aging

Another correctable medical cause for weight gain is the loss of muscle mass through inactivity or aging. This is usually a much slower process than the weight gain caused by serious organ diseases. As a person loses muscle, they often gain fat because muscle is our major calorie burner. Initially, there may be a negligible change in weight, but the body's shape will often change. The midline will expand with the accumulation of fat. Eventually most people will start to gain weight as they lose a significant amount of their muscle to burn up calories and their body fat adds up. This is a correctable problem. Just because a person is getting older does not mean they can't build up their muscles. The simple answer to this problem is weight-bearing exercises. This can be done at any point in our lives. More on this will be explained in chapter 5.

Finally, I want to reiterate that if you have an unexplained significant weight gain that occurs in a relatively short period of time, please first see your health-care provider to rule out any underlying medical condition that may be the source for those extra pounds.

CHAPTER

2

Basic Goals

For over forty years Canyon Ranch has been successful in helping people lose weight. The Canyon Ranch formula has not been complex. They simply remove individuals from their daily toxic living environment and place them in a safe, healthy, structured space. This eliminates those daily unhealthy temptations, like swinging by Starbuck's and grabbing a Frappuccino or having a beer or two with friends on the way home from work. Meals here at Canyon Ranch are served at certain scheduled times, and they don't serve food late at night. There is no big entertainment at night, so everyone goes to bed at a reasonable time, so they have the opportunity to get a good night's sleep. No, we can't all live in this wonderful healthy bubble that has been created at Canyon Ranch, but you can do the best you can to reproduce this type of environment.

As I alluded to in the introduction about Dr. Weil and the blood type diet, living a healthy structured life is crucial for one to attain and maintain wellness and be able to lose weight. This healthy structure is important in all facets of our lives. It includes how we sleep, eat, and work and when we exercise. Without structure our healthy lifestyles will fall through the cracks, and our ability to lose weight is significantly hindered.

Do your best to keep to a healthy routine. This is not to say there aren't going to be days when you fall out because of unforeseen events

33

that occur. For example, you may have to forgo your morning exercise because you were up half the night with a sick child, or friends may have come over to your house for dinner, and you ended up eating later than normal. The problem for many of us is that if something throws us off our regular routine, we may start sliding down the proverbial slippery slope, and the next thing we know is that all those bad habits start to return. When that happens the pounds you worked so hard to get rid of start to slowly creep back. The simple answer is if you are thrown a wrench onto your daily healthy routine, you need to accept it as a one-off, and on the next day go back to your regular salubrious lifestyle. Life is always going to throw a wrench, so simply accept it and get back on your horse. As I have told my child and my patients for years, when you have a perfect day, and everything goes right, this is actually the oddball day—not the normal day.

To help us maintain this healthy schedule, it's best to have routines that are reasonable and readily attainable. For example, if you decide you want to lose a lot of weight and do it quickly, you may decide you need to exercise for two hours every morning. To accomplish this great deed you have to get up two hours earlier than you normally do. Now you are getting two hours less sleep every night. It doesn't take long to realize that sleeping two hours less a night is making you more tired during the day. When this happens, as explained in the previous chapter about sleep disturbances, lack of sleep is a source of weight gain. After a while most people will start to feel that getting up two hours earlier is not worth it. In the end all your great plans to lose weight goes down the drain. Instead of setting up an unobtainable goal of getting up two hours earlier to work out, consider getting up an hour earlier than normal and possibly going to bed one hour earlier. Now that's something realistic, doable, and most importantly maintainable! That has been my philosophy for years.

Here are four very basic and attainable structural tasks we should all do daily to improve our health and weight loss:

1. Sleep well.
   ○ Get 7 to 9 hours of "good quality" sleep.
   ○ Go to bed and get up at the same time every day, even on weekends.

2. Schedule your eating time.
   (This plan assumes you don't work the night shift.)
   Eat meals at the same time each day within these parameters:
   ○ Breakfast 6 a.m. to 9 a.m.
   ○ Lunch: 11 a.m. to 1 p.m.
   ○ Dinner: 5 p.m. to 7 p.m.

3. Exercise moderately.
   You must exercise at least 150 minutes a week, and it must be spread out throughout the week at a scheduled time.

4. Meditate 10 minutes daily.

The specifics about what to do during those basic time periods will be addressed in future chapters.

Setting Realistic Numbers

If you have ruled out medical causes for weight gain, it's time to sit down and work on a game plan and determine what your goals are. My first goal for all my patients is not how much weight they can lose but how they can be healthier. As I have said, in the process of getting healthier, more often than not, a person will be able to lose those unwanted pounds. How do we know a person is healthy? Feeling well is a good first start in determining if you are healthy. The next step in evaluating how healthy you are is to look at certain biological numbers that need to be within a certain range to show that a person is in good health.

Let's start on the outside of our bodies and work our way inward. The first thing to check is a person's waist size. The reason this is so important is because in the midline region of our bodies, deep below our abdominal muscles, is a particular type of fat called visceral fat. It is the fat that surrounds our abdominal organs and can also be in our organs (for example, what we call "fatty liver disease"). It is well known that having too much fat increases a person's chances of having ill health. Specifically, having excess visceral fat has a high association with health maladies in the body. It is a major contributor to the development of chronic diseases like diabetes.

Visceral fat is different than hip fat, arm fat, or bottom fat. The difference is that visceral fat, unlike other fat in the body, is biologically active. It produces substances that can affect our health and has the potential of producing several substances that cause disease. It can manufacture angiotensin that causes arterial constriction and can elevate blood pressure. We have known for years that overweight people were at an increased risk for hypertension (high blood pressure), but we never knew why. Now we know. Many of the medications that we use to treat high blood pressure have been made to block the effects of angiotensin.[32] One such group is called ACE inhibitors. They are quite effective in lowering a person's blood pressure. A person who has excessive visceral fat and has high blood pressure can take an ACE inhibitor to lower their blood pressure. The other lifestyle non-pharmacologic approach is to lose visceral fat through a weight loss program. Often if this is accomplished, a person will not need to take a blood pressure medication or at the very least, be able to lower the dosage of the medication they are taking.

Another group of bioactive chemicals that are produced in the visceral fat are called cytokines.[33] Two specific types of cytokines are tumor necrosis factor alpha and interleukin-6. These chemicals are part of the immune system that can cause inflammation in the body. The body's production of these chemicals is typically elevated in diseases like rheumatoid arthritis, uncontrolled allergies, and asthma.

Since much of the pathogenesis of asthma is an inflammatory process, it is no wonder that the uptick in childhood asthma has mirrored the rise in childhood obesity.

Elevated visceral fat is commonly associated with an increased level of cholesterol in the body. This occurs because visceral fat releases free fatty acids into the portal vein. This vein directly empties its contents into the liver. It is the liver that makes approximately 60% of the bodies bad cholesterol called LDL. Therefore, individuals with excess visceral fat often have elevated LDL cholesterol levels.[34]

Finally, those individuals with excess visceral fat have the potential of developing insulin resistance. This means that your body's muscle and liver cells are less responsive to normal levels of insulin (the pancreatic hormone that carries glucose into the body's cells). There are two major mechanisms by which visceral obesity results in insulin resistance. The first appears to be related to the accumulation of fat in the liver that comes up the portal vein. This excess fat accumulation may result in impaired insulin signaling. The other potential cause of insulin resistance is through its production of inflammatory cytokines, which impairs insulin action.[35]

Since we know that excess visceral fat has the potential to cause ill health, we can measure waist size to estimate a person's level of visceral fat. When measuring a person's waist-size this is done at the level of the umbilicus (your belly button!), not under that midline protrusion. For men the waist size should be less than 38 inches, and for women it should be less than 35 inches. If the waist size is greater than these numbers, there is a high likelihood of elevated visceral fat.

The most accurate way to determine a person's quantity of visceral fat is to measure their body with a DEXA Scanner. (This is what we use at Canyon Ranch.) The advantage of this test is that it directly measures visceral fat. It is still an estimated amount of visceral fat, but this is much more accurate than only measuring waist size. By measuring visceral fat directly, it can explain the rare times when an overweight person does not have any of the metabolic complications associated with obesity, like high blood pressure, because they have little visceral fat. We refer to these individuals as the "overweight well individuals." I must reiterate that this is a rare person. By far, most people who are overweight, especially around their midline, have excess visceral fat.

Measuring visceral fat directly through a DEXA scanner also comes in handy with the skinny unwell person. They may have what would be considered nearly normal weight but unfortunately have excess visceral fat. When this happens, they are not in good health, and the visceral fat must be eliminated by improved lifestyle changes. This is another case that demonstrates that just because a person has gotten to a healthy weight does not necessarily mean they are healthy. That said, the far majority of overweight people have excess visceral fat and the normal or underweight person by far have a normal level of visceral fat.

Next, let's look at those goal numbers related to the prevention of cardiovascular disease, since it is still the number one killer of both men and women. One of the major risk factors for cardiovascular disease is an elevated blood pressure, also known as hypertension. So what numbers are considered to be high blood pressure? The acceptable numbers for normal blood pressure have lowered over the years. For years it was been generally accepted that a systolic (the top number) blood pressure above 140 was considered high blood pressure. This has been controversial over the past decade. There were many doctors that felt that this number was still too high, and they pushed to lower their patient's blood pressure to be less than 120 systolic. Fortunately, a very large study called the Sprint study[36] was performed to compare cardiovascular disease risk of those individuals who kept their systolic blood pressure under 140 versus those keeping it under

120. This study showed that there was less cardiovascular disease if people kept their systolic blood pressure lower than 120. For the bottom number, which is called your diastolic blood pressure, we like to see it less than 80 for decreased risk of cardiovascular disease.

It is interesting to note that at the time I was writing this book a new study re-evaluated the "Sprint" study and realized that the majority of participants with blood pressure in the 120s who were still having cardiovascular disease were women. There has been some preliminary conjecture that the ideal systolic BP for women may be lower than 120! This was noted in a study published in *Circulation Research* in February 2021 that looked at over 27,000 participants. The researchers of this study found that the risk of cardiovascular disease increased at the lower thresholds of systolic blood pressure for women. This disparity between women and men in their findings may be associated with differences in men's and women's cardiovascular anatomy and physiology. For instance, one major difference between men and women is that the diameter of women's arteries is smaller compared to men after normalizing the numbers for body size. At this time it's possible that the ideal systolic BP for women will be changed to a goal of less than 120. Stay tuned for potential important updates about what we have learned about blood pressure levels.

Another major risk factor for cardiovascular disease is cholesterol. There are several numbers on a cholesterol panel. The first is the total cholesterol number. Generally, we want this to be less than 200. It's important to note that total cholesterol is equal to the LDL, plus the HDL, plus one fifth of the triglycerides. It is for that reason that some people can have total cholesterol a little above 200 and their doctor may say there is nothing to worry about because their good cholesterol, the HDL, may be high. The LDL is called the bad cholesterol because its general job is to take cholesterol from the liver to the blood vessels where it can increase plaque build-up. I would like the LDL cholesterol to be less than 100 unless a person has known plaque (the stuff that clogs your arteries). If it is determined that you have plaque in your arteries, the LDL needs to be less than 70. This is based on the Jupiter study [37] that showed that if one has plaque in their arteries, there is a potential to have regression of that plaque if the LDL is less than 70. (There is another variable that also needs to be accomplished for plaque regression, and that is for your CRP, to be discussed shortly, to be less than 2.)

So how does one know if they are developing atherosclerosis (plaque)? Certainly, if an individual had a cardiovascular event like a heart attack or stroke, they have heart disease. Hopefully, it will be determined whether they have artery disease before that happens. One way to see if there is a buildup of plaque is by cardiac stress testing. The problem with that type of cardiac testing is that it doesn't begin to detect plaque formation until there is a critical obstruction in the arteries. It would be much better to determine if a person is forming plaque at an earlier stage.

One-way to see early plaque is to perform a CT calcium heart scan. This scan looks for calcifications in the coronary arteries, which indicates that a person has developed plaque. This is a good test for individuals over the age of 60. Under the age of 60 there are false negatives because it takes a period of time for calcium to collect in the arteries. A person younger than 60 may have plaque formation (called soft plaque) that has not yet calcified. For that reason I will advise my patients under the age of 60 to have a carotid ultrasound study. This picks up both non-calcified soft plaque and calcified plaque in your carotid arteries. If plaque is found, the goal for your LDL is to be less than 70. Otherwise the goal is to be less than 100mg/dl. It should be noted here that beyond the age of 60 the carotid ultrasound continues to be a good test and also does not produce the high dose radiation that is created by a CAT scan.

The goal numbers for high-density lipoprotein (HDL), the good cholesterol, is to be greater than 50 for women and greater than 40 for men. It plays a key role in prevention of atherosclerotic disease. It does this through various modalities. These include reverse cholesterol transport, which means removing excess cholesterol from macrophages at the level of the blood vessels and transporting that cholesterol to the liver where it is excreted in the bile or feces. HDL lowers oxidation and inflammation and improves endothelial function (arterial wall integrity) by increasing nitrous oxide (which is a vasodilator) and prevents cellular apoptosis (cell death).[38] It's a wonder pill in many ways.

Because of the many benefits of HDL, we often become complacent about the risks for cardiovascular disease if a person's HDL is extremely elevated. Very high levels of HDL may not be as protective against atherosclerosis as we originally thought. Studies have shown that there is a "U" shaped curve in the prevention of atherosclerosis as HDL levels elevate. In a study conducted by Dr. Marc Allard-Ratick, with Emory University School of Medicine in Atlanta, there were nearly 6000 participants whose average age was 63 and a third of the participants where women. They looked at HDL levels and found that the risk of having a heart attack or death from heart disease decreased as the HDL increased until it reached 60mg/dl. Beyond that level the protective effect of HDL decreased in a "U" shaped curve trajectory.[39] An example of this was a patient of mine who at the age of 64 had a high LDL of over 150 and a very high HDL of 115. Her primary care physician told her not to be concerned about her elevated LDL because her HDL was very high. Unfortunately she had a stroke at the age of 64. So the bottom line is that very high HDL levels may not be as protective as we originally thought.

So what is the formula for lowering cholesterol? The first thing is to improve a person's lifestyle with a low saturated fat diet and exercise. About 60% of a person's cholesterol level comes from the body's production of cholesterol and about 40% comes from the food they eat. This is somewhat of a misnomer because visceral fat is contributing factor in the production of LDL cholesterol. Therefore, if one has excess visceral fat and is able to lose it with improved lifestyles, it can have a significant impact on lowering a person's LDL level.

If a person does everything right and their LDL still remains elevated, they must consider medication. I've had patients who were quite frustrated because they had been on a very restrictive low-fat diet and still could not lower their cholesterol. These are the individuals that despite doing all the right things continued to manufacture excess cholesterol. When this happens the standard therapy is a statin. In general people don't like taking statins for an assortment of reasons. For some reason there has been a lot of negative press about these medications, especially in social media. Despite the fact that I live the Canyon Ranch lifestyle, my cholesterol has remained elevated. For that reason I, myself, take a statin medication. It hit home with me personally as I watched my father suffer from a major stroke and die at the age of 70, and my uncle who was even younger than me died of a stroke. Certainly, statins are far from a perfect drug and sometimes cause side effects. The most common unwanted reaction is muscle pain. Up to 10% of people taking statins complain of muscle pain. If a person has this problem, there are three basic options: stop the statin, try a different statin, or lower the dose of their present statin. When I choose a statin for my patients to take, I try to select one that is more hydrophilic, like rosuvastatin, rather than prescribing lipophilic statins. The statins that are more water-soluble than others don't seem to hang around in our system as long, and therefore appear to have fewer side effects.

Because these medicines are metabolized in the liver, there can be an occasional elevation of liver enzymes. This may mean there is a mild inflammation of the liver. Under the direction of your health-care provider, the statin dose may need to be adjusted or stopped all together. In addition, one has to be restrictive with certain foods such as grapefruit. Grapefruit competes with the enzyme that breaks down statins in the liver. In other words they both use the same enzyme to be metabolized. Because of this interaction, if a person ingests a grapefruit when they are taking a statin there is a potential of having an abnormally high concentration of the statin in their blood stream.

The most serious complication associated with statins is a condition called rhabdomyolysis. With this medical problem one can have actual muscle breakdown. This condition is extremely rare, and in all my years of practicing medicine I have not had one patient come down with this condition.

There has been a lot of negative information on the internet about statins. Much of it has to do with the perceived "evil" pharmaceutical companies. Yes, they are turning a profit, but they should for all the years of research they have done to make these potentially lifesaving drugs. I see patients all the time who come to see me as an integrative physician thinking I am going to give them some alternative therapy for a statin, such as an herbal alternative. If their numbers are not where they should be, and especially if there is evidence of cardiovascular disease, more often than not I will recommend taking a statin because they succeed in lowering cholesterol.

Another important biomarker is the C-reactive protein. This is a biomarker that measures the level of inflammation that is present in the body. The goal number is to be < 2 mg/L and ideally <1 mg/L (Be sure it is hs-CRP. HS stands for high sensitivity. This test can pick up very low levels of inflammation that is still associated with heart disease). It is a nonspecific test and does not identify the source of the inflammation. If the CRP is elevated, it only means there is an excess inflammatory process that is going on at that time. Some examples of inflammation are gingivitis, sinus infection, autoimmune diseases like rheumatoid arthritis, and excess visceral fat that produces cytokines. We now know that the formation of plaque in the arterial walls is often an active inflammatory process. Therefore, a person with excess inflammation in their body has an increased risk for having a heart attack or stroke. It is for that reason that I aggressively treat underlying inflammatory diseases like rheumatoid arthritis. This is done by recommending life-style changes and if necessary by prescribing medications.

It is well known that individuals who have diabetes and even pre-diabetes have an increased risk for other chronic diseases, such as cardiovascular disease and dementia. It is therefore important to aggressively treat diabetes and pre-diabetes by keeping their blood sugars under tight control. There are several goal numbers that need to be attained to show that a person's blood sugars are in the appropriate range. The first number is the fasting blood glucose level (the blood sugar reading before you have eaten anything in the morning). The goal is to be less than 100 mg/dl. Between 100 and 125 is considered pre-diabetic, and if it is greater than 125, that person can be considered a diabetic.

The next number to know is the hemoglobin A1C. This measures the percent of glucose that surrounds older red blood cells. Since the lifespan of a red blood cell is 90 days, this test helps determine how well a person's blood glucose has been controlled for the three months prior to the test being performed. Its reference range is 4.8% to 5.6%. If it is between 5.7% and 6.4% there is an indication that the person is pre-diabetic and above 6.5% a person can be considered a diabetic. It was originally used as a means to determine how well a diabetic controlled their blood sugars. At Canyon Ranch we use it as one of our diagnostic tools to look for diabetes and prediabetes.

Finally, the other test in relation to pre-diabetes is a fasting insulin level. The lab will give a reference range of 2mIU/L to 25mIU/L. If the number is greater than 15mIU/L, it tells me there is a higher risk that this person has insulin resistance. This means it takes more insulin to get glucose into the cells because of injury to insulin receptor sites on the surface of the cells. Increasing levels of insulin places a person at a higher risk of developing diabetes in the future.

The closer a person is to obtaining the numbers I have talked about in this chapter, the closer they are to being healthy.

Goal Numbers

1. **Cholesterol**
   - Total Cholesterol < 200mg/dl.
   - LDL Cholesterol < 100mg/dl unless there is plaque formation; then the number is <70mg/dl.
   - HDL Cholesterol > 50mg/dl for women and > 40mg/dl for men.

2. **Blood pressure**
   - < 120/80mm

3. **Blood sugars**
   - Fasting glucose < 100mg/dl
   - Fasting insulin < 15mlU/L
   - Hemoglobin A1C < 5.7%

4. **Inflammation**
   - C-Reactive Protein-hs < 2.0mg/L

5. **Body Fat**[40]
   - Women ages 18 to 49: goal 27 to 37%.
   - Women ages 50 to 84: goal 31 to 40% fat.
   - Men ages 18 to 49: goal 15 to 25% fat.
   - Men ages 50 to 84: goal 19 to 28% fat.

3

Our Metabolic Responses to Food

I often ask my patients what their health goals are for the coming year. For patients that are overweight, their answer is usually the number of pounds they would like to lose. It is a well-known scientific fact that being overweight increases the risk of many chronic diseases. Therefore, losing excess weight decreases a person's risk for future diseases. In addition, it can help control chronic diseases a person may have already developed. For example, diabetics who are able to lose weight often find that their blood sugars are much easier to control. They often need less, and sometimes no medication, to manage their diabetes.

However, it's important to know that losing weight is not the only goal we need to accomplish to improve our health. The type of diet and exercise we engage in to attain that goal may be unhealthy and often difficult to maintain. As I recounted in my introduction, my patient Jane was able to lose weight, but the particular diet she followed resulted in elevated cholesterol and placed her at a higher risk for cardiovascular disease. A better and more ideal scenario is for a person to first become metabolically healthy. In the process of attaining this goal, one will more often than not lose weight. When weight loss is performed this way, a person will be healthier, their risk for chronic disease is lowered, they have an increased potential for an expanded longevity and their quality of life improves.

So what do I mean when I say metabolically stable? It means that during the course of the day and night, markers of energy production and chemistries associated with the usage of these markers remain in the healthy range. If they consistently go above or below that range throughout the day, there is a higher risk for fat storage, inflammation, and increased oxidative stress. This can ultimately cause weight gain and increase the risk for chronic disease.

Over the years, the medical establishment has assumed that everyone's metabolic response to food was the same. One such example is our use of the glycemic index. We have used this index to determine how fast certain carbs are broken down to glucose and enter into the blood stream. We have known for a long time that simpler carbs tend to break down into glucose and enter the blood stream much faster than complex carbs. The more rapidly a carb is broken down to its simple sugar, glucose, the greater the risk is for weight gain. The glycemic index was developed by using a large cohort of all kinds of individuals to measure the average time it takes to breakdown carbohydrates to glucose into the blood stream.

Therefore the glycemic index assumes that the length of time it takes for a food to go from a whole food to glucose in the blood would be the same for everyone. This is okay if you are the average individual and your metabolic response to food is in the center of the sampling bell curve. The problem of course is that not everyone sits in the middle of the bell curve. So what about the individuals on either side of the bell curve? Their metabolic response to foods will vary.

The general public has known for years that we are all very different in how we metabolize food. How many times have you heard from someone that one particular individual can eat all they want and not gain an ounce and another person can just look at the same food and seem to gain 10 pounds? Well, the Weizmann Clinic in Israel decided to look at this and see what was up. They took 800 people and gave them 50,000 meals. During each meal the participants would all eat the same thing. Immediately after eating they measured each individual's blood glucose, insulin and triglyceride and followed their responses over a finite period of time.[41] What they found out was quite surprising. Many had similar responses to foods, but many responses were very different, even for identical twins! So we are different after all!

The Weizmann Study has been reproduced in the Predict Study.[42] It had a larger number of participants over a longer period of time. In this study they started off with 1100 individuals. It began in 2018 and they now have over 10,000 individuals in the study. This study confirmed what the Weizmann Study previously showed. The Predict study then took it a little further and attempted to determine what the variables were that caused the difference in metabolic responses to foods among individuals. Those variables were:

- **Meal composition:** This means a person's metabolic response to what they eat can be affected by all the other foods they consume during that meal or snack. Therefore, by adding certain proteins or healthy fats to a meal, you can affect the absorption of the food you are eating.

- **A person's age, sex, and weight.** These can all affect food absorption.

- If a person has any **disease or inflammation** in the body, it can change a person's metabolic response.

- The type of bacteria in a person's gut, called their **gut microbiome**, can affect the metabolic response.

- A person's **genetics**. It has been shown that identical twins have a closer response to foods than fraternal twins. (However it is important to note that even identical twins can have different metabolic responses.)

- **Meal timing:** This will be discussed in detail later. The time you eat your meal during the day can be almost as important as what you eat.

- ○ **Sleep:** A person's quantity and quality of sleep can affect their metabolic response to food.

- ○ A person's **emotional state:** For example, if a person is stressed, they can produce excessive amounts of the stress hormone, cortisol, which can affect their body metabolically.

In doing research, clinical data can be obtained by doing things like placing an intravenous port in a person's vein for easy access for blood testing throughout the day. For the general public this is cumbersome and nearly impossible to carry out. Fortunately the technology for this has improved, and we now have devices that do not need an intravenous port. One of these devices is a continuous glucose monitor (CGM). Diabetics have used these for several years. At Canyon Ranch we use the Abbott freestyle Libre CGM to measure a person's glucose for two weeks. This device utilizes a very small filament that is placed in the subcutaneous tissues and remains there so that it continuously measures a person's glucose.

It is important to note that there is a short lag of time from what a person's actual blood glucose is to what is measured by the filament that is placed in the subcutaneous tissue. Measuring a person's glucose on a continuous basis not only tells us what a person's glucose level is but based on the glucose readings, gives a pretty good idea about what is happening with the person's blood insulin level. Insulin's job is to take glucose from the blood stream and put into the cell to be utilized for energy. Therefore, insulin will proportionately respond to the amount of glucose that is in the blood stream.

To interpret the numbers that are produced by the glucose monitor, it's important to know what a normal blood glucose response to foods should be. The normal measurement for a fasting glucose (first morning blood sugar, before any food or drink is ingested) is less than 100mg/dl. If the glucose reading consistently measures between

100mg/dl and 125mg/dl, this is considered pre-diabetic. If the fasting blood sugar is consistently above 125mg/dl, the person would be considered a diabetic. If a person's fasting blood sugars are consistently elevated, they should discuss this with their health-care provider to prevent future health problems.

For the non-diabetics a normal metabolic response to food will not have a glucose elevation above 140mg/dl. If there is a rapid incline of a person's glucose level above 140 after eating, the body will respond by generating a significant rapid production of insulin. When there is an exaggerated over-production of a person's insulin, it can cause unwanted physiologic responses. Those unwanted responses are:

○ **Storage of Fat**.

○ An increase in **inflammation** in the body.

○ A potential for **injury to the lining of blood vessel walls**.

○ Can **increase oxidase stress** (this the production of cell damaging free radicles in the body that increases chronic disease risk).

A cycle of repeated spiking of glucose will result in a corresponding spiking of insulin. The upshot of these metabolic changes is often weight gain. However, please don't panic if you eat an occasional cookie. Weight gain comes from the repeated spikes in glucose and insulin. However, if one cookie leads to another cookie on a regular basis, that is different story.

As we have learned, if there is a significant rapid spike in your blood glucose, there is a corresponding spike in insulin. This spike in insulin does exactly what it should do and causes a rapid drop in the body's glucose. But sometimes it overshoots the baseline and causes true hypoglycemia. Or because there is a significant drop in glucose the body thinks it is hypoglycemic (a relative hypoglycemia). Because the brain requires a constant supply of blood glucose, if you are hypoglycemic or are rapidly dropping in your amounts of blood sugar, this will stimulate the adrenal glands to release two hormones called adrenaline and cortisol. These two hormones then signal the liver to convert the stored carbohydrates, called glycogen, into glucose and release it into the bloodstream.

Most of us know how hypoglycemia feels. The symptoms produced by adrenaline are similar to the feelings we get when we are anxious. We can experience nervousness, sweating, faintness, a fast heartbeat, tingling, nausea, and trembling. In addition, if the brain can't get enough glucose, we may feel weak, dizzy, tired, drowsy, confused, and have a sensation of peril. Have you noticed what we generally do when we feel this way? Without our thinking, our bodies tell us what to do. We immediately start scavenging around for something sweet to eat. As a result, not only do we potentially gain weight when our insulin spikes. We often eat more food, and eat the wrong foods, after our blood sugar drops.

The likely culprits causing a spike in a person's blood glucose are the carbohydrates consumed during the meal. The less complex a carbohydrate is, the more likely it is to cause a spike in glucose. Some less complex carbohydrate examples are foods like pancake syrup or soft drinks. If you are not eating obvious simple carbohydrates, you should start looking for other carbs like potatoes or breads. It's not always that easy to find the carb source for the spike, especially if you ate the same carb previously in a meal and had no spike. If that happens, the next thing you need to look at is the meal's composition. Certain proteins or fats can slow down the absorption of the carbs and result in little or no spike.

I saw an example of this in my personal glucose readings from what I was eating for breakfast. My three days of readings are shown below (see figure 1). As you can see, on Day 1, I ate granola, blueberries, and unsweetened almond milk. With this breakfast I spiked my sugar to 171mg/dl (As stated previously a glucose spike greater than 140 is a concern.). On day 2, right before eating, I went for a one-hour bike ride. I ate the same breakfast, but because I had exercised, I burnt up some of the calories, causing my post-meal glucose spike to be less at 152mg/dl. On Day 3, instead of having the same breakfast I had on the two previous days, I ate only eggs for breakfast and did not exercise. As you can see in the chart below, this resulted in no glucose spike. So the simple solution seemed to be to eat more eggs and look for a cereal that doesn't contain honey or eat my berries with a meal that contains more protein.

I certainly don't want to be like my patient Jane who eats only eggs for breakfast. I might lose weight, but my cholesterol level would likely elevate. This is not a good thing for a person who has a strong family history of cardiovascular disease. Because I had my device in, I was able to experiment with my breakfast meal and create a healthy breakfast that wouldn't cause a spike in my glucose and at the same time would not increase my risk for cardiovascular disease.

Glucose Readings from My Breakfast Meals

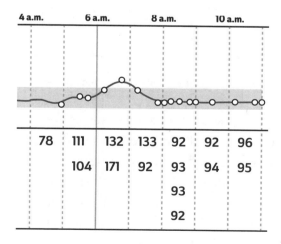

4 a.m.	6 a.m.		8 a.m.		10 a.m.	
78	111	132	133	92	92	96
	104	171	92	93	94	95
				93		
				92		

Day 1: Granola cereal with unsweetened almond milk and blueberries and no exercise

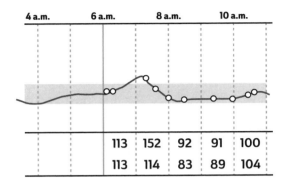

		4 a.m.	6 a.m.	8 a.m.	10 a.m.	
		113	152	92	91	100
		113	114	83	89	104

Day 2: Granola with unsweetened almond milk, blueberries and 1-hour bike ride

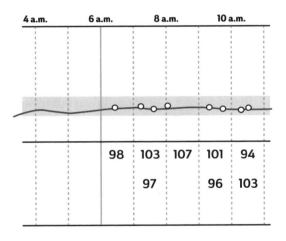

		4 a.m.	6 a.m.	8 a.m.	10 a.m.	
		98	103	107	101	94
			97		96	103

Day 3: Egg omelet with cheese and no exercise

Other common sources of glucose spikes are juices and smoothies. In the case of juices this is a no brainer. When one squeezes out the fruit juice, it contains highly concentrated sugar and there is little or no fiber to slow down its absorption. The result is a spike in glucose. Smoothies fool many of us. Everyone thinks that when you concentrate and jam all those healthy fruits and vegetables in one tall glass it has to be good and healthy for us. But at times it can be a problem.

Don't get me wrong. More often than not your smoothie may contain boatloads of vitamins and antioxidants that the body needs and loves to help prevent disease. However, if one is trying to lose weight, a concentrated liquid from several sugar-laden foods has the potential of causing a glucose spike in the blood stream. When you break down and blend all those ingredients, the time that it takes to metabolize the food to glucose is significantly shortened compared to eating the whole unblended foods. The final result is often that many of these "healthy" smoothies cause an increased risk for blood glucose spikes, which in turn produces an insulin spike that increases the risk for weight gain.

At this point you may be thinking that carbs must be the evil enemy, and all those meat-eating Keto dieters were right after all. Well, certainly you are realizing why the Keto diet is affective for weight loss. Without eating carbs one does not get spikes in their glucose and subsequently will not have spikes in their insulin. But, as you will learn in chapter 8, a true Keto diet has a lot of potentially unhealthy aspects associated with it. As I said at the beginning of this book, a person's endpoint in a diet and exercise program is to be healthier, and in the process of getting healthier, you can lose weight.

Designing a diet around a person's metabolic response to food gives them a more personalized approach to their diet. I know many of you who live in a home with more than one person may be thinking that there is no way you can cook or prepare food separately for each individual in the household. However, one must first realize that being overweight is a very serious health issue that can lead to many chronic illnesses. Making a little effort to eliminate a risk of causing this will be paid off many times over. The cost, let alone the morbidity and mortality of chronic disease, is astronomical. The relatively small effort to make adjustments to having foods we should eat is more than worth it. In addition, the actual practical aspect of proceeding with this program is not as difficult as one would think.

4

Meal Timing, and Do We Need to Eat Breakfast?

Over the years the only treatment plan prescribed by most physicians for losing weight was a simple 1200 or 1500 calories diet that was handed out to the patient at the time of their office visit. I must sadly confess to practicing this so-called treatment plan for much of the first half of my professional career. This numeric diet plan gave a person the total number of calories they were allowed to eat in a day. The assumption was made that if they only ate those calories or less per day, they would lose weight. There was little focus on when those calories were to be ingested. It was only important to not eat more than the number of calories allotted. Most people that followed this calorie counting diet ingested those calories when it was most convenient for them. In most homes this was at the end of the day. People would save up those food calories during the day because they were too busy to eat or were not exceptionally hungry during the day. Many would take it to an extreme and practically starve themselves all day so they could eat their big meal at the end in the evening. This was not that hard because the typical American diet traditionally encourages us to have a large meal at supper time.

In addition to societal pressures to eating a big meal when the day ends, there are physiological reasons that reinforce this habit. One reason is that it was found that ghrelin levels are higher during the evening than during the morning. Ghrelin is the hormone that is produced and released mainly by the stomach with smaller amounts released by the small intestine, pancreas, and brain. Ghrelin stimulates our appetite, increases food intake and promotes fat storage. That is one of the main reasons for our basic need to eat the bulk of our food at the end of the day.

As the science of weight loss continues to advance, we are learning that when we eat can be almost as important as what we eat. Food timing has become an emerging science as it relates to weight gain and weight loss. When we eat can affect us in terms of weight loss almost as much as the quantity of food ingested during specific mealtimes.

One of the strongest scientific evidences related to food timing and weight gain was seen if a person consistently eats lunch after 3 p.m. It has been shown that late lunch eaters (after 3 p.m.) lost less weight during an experimental treatment group than early lunch eaters (before 3 p.m.), in spite of having similar age, appetite hormones, energy intake and expenditure, sleep duration, and macronutrients distribution.[43]

How you spread your calories out during the day can also affect your ability to lose weight. This was seen in another study done by Jakubowicz et. al. It was shown that those subjects assigned to a small breakfast and a large dinner lost significantly less weight than those assigned to a large breakfast and a small dinner. The science behind this is that our peak sensitivity to glucose is at noon. After this time our sensitivity decreases as the day goes on. The later a person eats after 12:00 noon, the less is the person's sensitivity to glucose. What this means is that a person needs to produce more insulin later in the day for the same type and quantity of food they may have eaten earlier in the day. Indeed, a 12-week experimental study in overweight women with metabolic syndrome (a prediabetic state) randomized into two groups. Both ate the same total number of calories, but one group ate most of their calories at the beginning of the day and the other ate most of their calories at the end of the day. The subjects that ate the largest caloric intake during dinner had a higher level of insulin resistance than those with the largest caloric intake during breakfast. Because of that, the later in the day caloric consumers had a much more difficult time losing weight.[44]

The hormone melatonin is an additional factor that can affect food timing. Melatonin has long been known as a sleep aid that helps a person fall sleep. It is commonly sold at pharmacies and health stores. Melatonin is a hormone known for its central role in the circadian system (the 24-hour cycle). It signals the brain and body that it is nighttime, and it is time to get ready for bed. This allows us to go to bed at a respectable time and helps us fall asleep. The effect that melatonin can have on our weight is that it can affect glucose metabolism. It has been shown that melatonin may worsen glucose intolerance.[45] This causes an increased production of insulin to mobilize glucose into the cells compared to those people that ate earlier. Once again, remember that higher productions of insulin can potentially increase fat storage.

The numbers are very convincing. Eating large high-energy foods during the two hours before bedtime increases five times the probability of being obese. Among those individuals who have a higher food intake within two hours after waking up, have lower odds of being obese and double the probability of having a healthy weight.[46] Another way of looking at this is that one should try to have a long-time difference between caloric midpoint (average time at which 50% of daily calories are consumed) and the onset of melatonin production, which is ½ hour prior to bedtime.

Geneticists are beginning to learn that there are certain individuals who have a particular genetic makeup that makes them more susceptible to the effects of meal timing and melatonin. In the future we may be able indicate who can be affected by eating a later meal and who can't. This is the essence of a truly personalized medicine approach to our health. Until this is totally ironed out, we will need to treat everyone the same on this and advise anyone who is trying to lose weight to not eat late at night.

There has long been a general understanding among most people that the idea of eating a big dinner late at night probably is not a good idea. Even though this has long been a pervasive view among the masses, we have a hard time admitting it. There are so many social implications associated with this. Who doesn't want to gather around a big meal at the end of the day with family and friends or go out for dinner and celebrate surviving another day? We have been socially ingrained to have that big meal at the end of the day. However, if you ask most people if they think it's a healthy thing to stuff ourselves with a large meal at the end of the day, most will say no. But since there is safety in numbers along with all the joy that's wrapped up in that big evening meal, we still do it.

With all the science that is right in front of our faces about the potential negative outcomes that can result from eating late, mainly weight gain, we have to rethink the evening meal. If you are serious about losing weight, you must learn to not be top heavy with the majority of your caloric intake during your evening meal. Lunch must be a larger meal compared to dinner, and it must be eaten before 3:00 p.m. You must have your evening meal early in the evening to be sure you are eating it at a time when insulin will be more effective compared to eating late in the evening.

Even though most of us eat our biggest meal at the end of the day, the majority of us realize that it's probably not a great idea. This is not controversial for most of us; we just need to make the change. Our real debate is about breakfast. Do we really need to eat breakfast when many of us aren't that hungry in the morning? Invariably when I am lecturing to a group of guests at Canyon Ranch, someone in the audience will ask if they must eat breakfast. At that point everyone in the audience will turn their heads toward me to hear what my answer is. For years as children we listened to our mothers and fathers at the breakfast table saying, "Breakfast is the most important meal of the day, so you are not getting up from the breakfast table until you have finished all your breakfast!"

But do we really need to have breakfast, especially if we are trying to lose weight? The intermittent fasting crowd readily answers no. It seems to be the easiest meal in the day to skip for a variety of reasons—social, situational, time, and so forth—or we give the main reason many of us don't want to eat breakfast. We just aren't hungry in the morning. There have been many theories about why many of us don't eat breakfast. Most of these theories are based around our hormones that affect our appetites. Leptin, which suppresses our appetite secretes in a diurnal rhythm, has its lowest levels of the day in the morning. On the surface, this would seem to make us want us to eat less in the morning. However, an interesting large-scale study of over 5,000 participants called the NHAES III study showed that even though leptin levels for most individuals is lowest in the a.m., those that skipped breakfast on the whole had 50% greater blood levels of leptin which decreases their appetite. Therefore those individuals that had the highest levels of the food suppressing hormone leptin in the mornings were those people most likely to skip breakfast.[47]

The numbers of people skipping breakfast is pretty staggering. Based on a national survey, approximately one quarter of American adults skip breakfast. About half of young adults report that they are "too rushed in the morning to eat a healthy breakfast." There are socio-demographic and lifestyle factors that are associated with those that skip breakfast. These factors include younger age, poverty, African

American race, male sex, lower education, non-Southern regions of the United States of America, urban residence, smokers, alcohol use, and infrequent exercise.[48]

As you can see from this list, those that skip breakfast have a higher correlation with unhealthy behaviors, such as smoking and alcohol consumption poorer diets, and lower physical activity. They also tend to have a higher metabolic risk, that is, a higher body mass index (BMI), larger waist circumference, higher fasting insulin, and increased cholesterol and LDL levels than those individuals that don't skip breakfast.[49]

Additional studies show a relationship between eating breakfast and having a decreased appetite and increased satiety throughout the rest of the day compared to those who do not eat breakfast. Daily ghrelin (the hormone in the body that increases hunger) production was reduced and daily fullness was increased for those who ate breakfast compared with those who skipped breakfast.[50]

Another interesting study performed by Leidy et al. completed a 12-wk RCT (random controlled trial) in 57 breakfast-skipping adolescents (age: 19 ± 1 y; BMI: 29.7 ± 4.6) who were provided with one of 3 types of breakfast: (1) higher-protein breakfasts, (2) normal-protein breakfasts or (3) continued skipping of breakfast. Baseline and post-study assessments of hourly hunger and fullness were collected. The consumption of breakfast, particularly the higher-protein versions, led to reductions in daily hunger compared with skipping breakfast; however, the normal-protein breakfast did not result in a lessening of hunger.[51]

What happens when instead of eating a breakfast we have one of those morning "healthy" meal replacement beverages? Many of us do it. We simply throw a healthy premade powder, some berries, and almond or soy milk into a blender and off we go. Perhaps we've had instant breakfasts for years. Many of us gulp down what we think is a reduced-calorie liquid diet for weight loss. However, when compared with solid foods, many of these beverages elicit a weaker satiety effect and a greater subsequent energy intake, possibly due to the faster digestive and absorptive rates of beverages. Of 22 studies of breakfast meals reviewed, 5 included beverage breakfasts. The beverage meals led to a minimal to no effect on postprandial hunger and fullness compared with the solid or mixed meals. When the studies containing beverage meals were removed, the impact of breakfast consumption on appetite and satiety strengthened compared with breakfast skipping. Collectively, the evidence supports the inclusion of solid foods at breakfast to elicit improvements in appetite control and satiety.[52]

So it comes down to the fact that eating breakfast may not be "the" most important meal of the day, but it appears to have a modest effect in helping in weight management as long as it contains a high content of solid food protein and is not a beverage (smoothie-type). Those who are faithful to your morning health shake, especially those who have your smoothie-blended marvel with everything in it, including healthy kale, muscle building proteins, and great antioxidants, please don't fret. The magical concoction you love to drink right after your morning run may still be okay to consume as long as you monitor your blood sugars after consuming this. As discussed in the previous chapter, you can experiment with different breakfast smoothies and determine what combination of fiber and other ingredients causes the least spike or no glucose spike.

Lastly, one of the most important studies that looked at individuals who were able to lose weight and keep it off has been the National Weight Control Registry. (More will be discussed about the NWR in the chapter on weight loss maintenance.) There are over 10,000 individuals in this group. To be in this study group a person must have lost at least 30 pounds and kept it off for more than one year. The average person in the group has lost 66 pounds and kept it off for greater than 5.5 years. In this successful weight-losing group, 78% of them ate breakfast. [53] With such a high percent of breakfast eaters among very successful long-term weight loss individuals, this alone is very convincing evidence to recommend a daily non-smoothie, high protein breakfast to help lose weight.

5

We Must Exercise to Lose Weight. It's Non-Negotiable.

It is common for many of us to make changes in our diets to improve our health and to help us lose weight. Those of us that want to lose that extra layer know they have to make some type of dietary changes to allow this to happen. However, when it comes to exercise to lose weight, many of us see it as an insurmountable barrier that we don't want to take on. We hear our friends talking about joining gyms and working out five days a week before or after work. It seems so overwhelming that there is no desire to attempt it. But here is the cold reality. If you are serious about losing weight, want to improve your quality of life and potentially increase your lifespan, you have to exercise. Exercising regularly is non-negotiable!

The simple fact is that in a person's quest to lose weight, they eat fewer calories. Unfortunately, when we eat fewer calories, our bodies go into survival mode. The body thinks it's going to starve. Therefore the body's natural reaction is to slow down its metabolism so it doesn't burn up as many calories. Even though a person is eating less, they may not be able lose weight unless they exercise. To keep from going into starvation mode and prevent the body's metabolism from slowing down, a person has to exercise.

In addition to preventing our metabolism from slowing down, exercise has many other health benefits. There is not a medication in my physician pharmacopeia that can touch what exercise can do for us for keeping us healthy. Exercise can do the following:

- Keeps a person's metabolism from slowing down when they ingest fewer calories

- Helps lower blood pressure. This is accomplished by slowing down the resting heart rate and dilating blood vessels.

- Lowers LDL (the "Bad" cholesterol).

- Increases HDL (the "Good" cholesterol).

- Lowers inflammation. The biomarker for inflammation, CRP, has been shown to be lower with regular exercise.

- Makes us more sensitive to insulin if we exercise regularly. More insulin sensitivity means less overall need for insulin, which as explained in the metabolism chapter 3, decreases fat storage, inflammation, and hunger.

- Helps lower our stress levels. With less stress there is less excess production of the stress hormone, cortisol, which mobilizes fats and increases abdominal weight gain.

In many ways exercise is the miracle "drug!" If you are truly serious about weight loss and improving your health, you need to exercise. If I'm slowly convincing you that you must exercise, what kind of exercise should you do and how long should you perform it? These are important questions. Let me start here by telling you a little secrete. I personally don't like to exercise. My favorite time of exercising is when I finish my exercise. I don't enjoy getting out of bed at 5:00 a.m.

getting my cycling gear on, and then climbing on my bike and taking off for an hour. I don't really like to go to the gym after work 2 or 3 days a week to weight train. I always have to go through some self-talk to get myself to do it. I have many friends who, unlike me, love to exercise. They can't wait to go for a run or throw some weights high into the air. That is not me. I do it for all the reasons I've pointed out. It's non-negotiable. Not only do I do it to keep my weight off and improve my overall health; I do it because it makes me feel good. This feeling of well-being is very difficult to define. If, for various reasons such as family issues or excess work or travelling, I am unable to exercise for several days in a row, I find I feel tired and draggy. My mood seems to change, and I don't have that daily happy spark about me.

So what is a good exercise program? It all depends on where you are starting from and how far are you willing to go. For some individuals a good exercise program is simply getting up and walking a mile or so about 3 days a week. That's a great beginning and starts the march towards a healthier you. Actually, any movement in which you are getting your heart rate up is good movement to start with. It does not need to be a formalized structured program at first. Certainly, there is no need to run a marathon to be healthy. If it takes baby steps to get you moving, then that is absolutely fine. The most difficult aspect of any exercise program is committing to it and doing it. It is often easier to continue an exercise program than it is to begin an exercise program.

If you are interested in a more personalized approach to an exercise program, it is best to start out by knowing your body composition. This is an important first step in customizing an exercise regime. For example, if after obtaining a person's body composition it is found that under all that unwanted adipose tissue is a warehouse of muscle, this individual should not be spending the majority of their precious time pounding weights in the weight room. The bulk of their time should be used to employ those wonderful muscles in burning up calories by doing cardio exercises like running or biking.

The gold standard for obtaining a person's body composition is a DEXA body scanner. This is what we use here at Canyon Ranch. This can accurately tell a person's percentage of body fat and how much lean mass (which is predominately muscle mass) they have. Many bathroom scales give a percentage of body fat. But one must know that it is not nearly as accurate as a DEXA scanner, and it often underestimates a person's body fat.

In order to determine if you have enough muscle to burn up those unwanted calories and you do not have access to a DEXA scanner that can directly measure your lean (nonfat) mass, you can estimate the amount of muscle mass by first obtaining your body fat percent by using various devices. The bathroom scales that measure percent body fat and a handheld devise found at most fitness facilities both utilize electrical impedance that will give you an estimate of percent body fat. With this information you can then use the following formula: Multiply your percent of body fat by your total weight, and that will give you the number of pounds of body fat you have. Lean mass is everything that is not fat or bone. That includes muscle (the far majority) and organs. Therefore the difference of the body fat from a person's total weight is their lean mass plus bone weight. Bone weight is really not much. For women it is about 5 to 6 pounds and for men about 6 to 7 pounds. So take that into consideration when you are calculating your lean mass.

To know whether or not a person has enough muscle to burn up those excess calories, women should have at least 90 pounds of lean mass, and men should have at least 130 pounds. If a person has low lean mass, they need to first focus on weight training to build up muscle before they begin any type of caloric restriction or excessive cardio exercises. The last thing one wants to do is to lose more muscle mass if they are trying to lose weight. Remember, muscles are the calorie burning machines of the body.

If it is determined that you need to work on building up muscle first in your exercise program, the best way to know how to properly do weight training is to work with a personal trainer or an exercise physiologist. They will show the proper way to efficiently build muscles and at the same time keep you from getting hurt. One must remember that this is not a sprint. One needs to take their time and slowly increase their weight training time and the amount of weight resistance. A good initial goal is to do some form of weight-bearing exercise 2 to 3 days a week. When you feel that you have build-up a significant amount of muscle, then is the time to increase your cardiovascular workout and have a more restrictive diet. Of course if you start out with adequate muscles mass, then it is okay to start your cardiovascular workout and dietary restrictions from the beginning.

There are many different cardiovascular exercises. They include fast walking, running, cycling, swimming or working out on a rowing machine. To be considered an effective cardiovascular exercise, it needs to be performed at an intensity in which a person's heart rate is between 70 and 85% of their predicted heart rate (220 minus a person's age equals their predicted heart rate). To maintain their current physical health state a person needs to exercise a minimum of 3 days a week for at least 30 minutes per workout. To improve a person's health and help them lose weight, it should be 5 days a week. I must point out here that in the beginning if someone, because of time restraint or being deconditioned, can walk only 3 days a week and their heart rate is not elevating into the target zone please don't give up. The inertia is moving in the right direction. In time to lose weight the goal is to exercise 5 days a week with adequate intensity for at least 30 to 60 minutes.

I want to briefly mention High Intensity Interval Training (HIIT). This type of workout is the most difficult but the most efficient.

Essentially a HIIT workout is doing a cardio exercise that a person increases the intensity of their exercise at intervals throughout the workout above that 85% predicted maximum heart rate. The advantage of this type workout is a person burns up a significantly higher number of calories compared to a regular cardio exercise. It certainly is not as much fun to exercise when one undertakes a HIIT program but if one wants to maximize their exercise time they should consider doing this type of exercise program.

The bottom line is that you have to move. Generally, the more you exercise, the easier it is to lose weight. However, I must caution you to gradually increase your exercise program. The last thing you want to do is hurt yourself by straining a muscle or getting tendonitis from overdoing it. When that happens you have to stop your exercise program and wait till it heals. A gradually increasing exercise program is the smart path to excellent health.

The last thing I must say about undertaking an exercise program, especially if you have not exercised much in the past, is to be sure to see your physician and be cleared to exercise. Your doctor can rule out any underlying cardiovascular maladies that may limit your exercise program—especially if you are considering doing HIIT type of workouts.

6

Changing Bad Habits

Because we are humans, we all have some bad habits. Some of these habits are worse to our health than others. What constitutes a truly bad habit changes as our scientific knowledge advances and societal values evolve over time. Growing up in the 1950s and 1960s, smoking tobacco was not really considered a bad habit. In fact it was portrayed as chic, and almost everyone in the movies smoked. Both my parents smoked, and all their friends smoked. It was a sign you were now an adult when you "learned" to smoke. For decades, drinking alcohol has been considered a sign of sophistication with actors drinking on TV commercials, shows, and in movies. We all know that drinking alcohol in excess can be a serious and even life-threatening bad habit. How do we judge when a habit becomes a bad or unhealthy habit? The simple answer is that if you are doing something repeatedly that is causing, or could cause ill health, it can be considered a bad habit.

There are many habits that are probably not a good thing to keep doing. And other habits must be stopped ASAP because they have obvious harmful effects. The first in this group of non-negotiable must-stop-now bad habit is smoking. There is no place for smoking if you want to be healthy. There is absolutely nothing good about a habit of smoking cigarettes. It is the primary source of many cancers such as lung and bladder cancer. It is a major cause of heart disease and strokes and is the number one cause of debilitating chronic lung disease, which includes emphysema and chronic bronchitis.

Many smokers don't want to quit because their biggest fear is if they stop smoking, they will gain weight. That is a real concern, but there is no good reason to risk the damage cigarettes can cause in our lives, period. It doesn't take an Einstein to recognize that if a person quits one oral pleasure, they'll want to replace it with another oral delight. The most likely replacement is food. Knowing this fact is a potential problem is the first step in dealing with this dilemma. There are a few things that can prevent people from replacing smoking with food. The next step should be to avoid those times and places where you usually did your smoking; for example, the smoking chair in front of the TV after dinner. Instead of sitting in that chair, go for a walk after dinner. Another easy tool I have advised my patients to do over the years is rather than grabbing a cigarette to put in your mouth, suck on a cinnamon stick. Fortunately I have never been a smoker, so the idea of sucking on a cinnamon stick doesn't sound too exciting. However, my patients have told me the particular taste of a cinnamon stick and being able to be able to roll the stick around in their fingers like people often do with a cigarette rather miraculously seems to satisfy their desire to have a cigarette. If you have gained 5 or more pounds after quitting smoking, it is time to go on high alert and stop this downward spiral now. Talk to your physician or a therapist to work on a game plan to prevent further weight gain and hopefully turn things around to start losing weight.

When people started to come out of their caves with the lessening of the Covid-19 pandemic, many realized they had two problems. The first was weight gain. There were many reasons for this weight gain, one of which was a lack of exercise. Many people before the outbreak of the deadly coronavirus got their exercise by going to the gym every day. As we know, most gyms were closed at that time. Another reason for weight gain was the excessive stress experienced by individuals dealing with the many traumas that resulted from the pandemic. People lost friends, family members, and many lost their jobs. The body's response to all this stress is the production of the stress hormone, cortisol. Cortisol is helpful for our survival in life-threatening situations. This hormone mobilizes fats and sugars to give us fuel to help us deal with a potential threat. If the stress we have is not finite but is ongoing, the movement of fats and surplus blood sugar manufactured from the overproduction of cortisol will in time add pounds to our bodies.

The other major source of weight gain during the pandemic was overeating. People were at home doing their Zoom meetings and they had time to cook large meals that were not necessarily healthy. Every time I personally got on a Zoom meeting it seemed like somebody in the group had a new recipe, and the biggest hit was usually sourdough bread.

The other big problem that occurred for many during sheltering at home was an increased consumption of alcohol. Most people who increased their alcohol consumption would never call themselves an alcoholic. However, with so much time spent at home instead of traveling to the office, it was too easy to pop a cold one earlier and earlier in the day. There was little concern about drinking and driving because we didn't go anywhere during the pandemic. In addition to having a drink or two on Friday or Saturday night after a long week of work, many started to have a cocktail on Thursday, then Wednesday. In addition, since many were confined with their partners, they were entertaining each other and sharing a bottle of wine in the middle of the week. In the past, one partner might not normally have a drink, but during the pandemic they began to join their partner for this mutually shared event. This ritual turned from having an occasional drink together to having two or three alcoholic drinks every night. I heard a similar story of this over and over again with many of my patients.

They are not alcoholics but were certainly drinking much more than they had in the past. It is important to remember that alcohol has 7 calories per gram, whereas sugar has only 4. One of the reasons people drink is because it decreases their inhibitions and relaxes them. So when that happens, that little voice that normally says, "Don't eat those potato chips or cheese before dinner" has left the room.

People often drink alcohol to help them fall asleep. However after about three hours of sleep, the alcohol causes a rebound alertness that often results in the person waking up. To make things worse they commonly have a very difficult time falling back to sleep. All this produces poor sleep. As discussed earlier, not getting good sleep can increase one's appetite the next day. And then guess who is suddenly eating a jelly donut the next morning.

How we attack our bad habits is very individualistic. Some people want to stop all alcohol, quit smoking, start exercising the next day, and eat a pristine perfect diet. For others the big first move may be to cut from three glasses of wine at night to two glasses. We need to know who we are, and what we can do, and what we are willing to do. The bottom line is you have to do something. Whether it's a giant leap or a baby step, we have to move forward to make improvements. What I have found in my years of practicing medicine and what the studies have shown is that those who decide themselves that they need to make changes to be more healthy are more successful in this than having a friend or a family member or coworker push them to change their routines. Many of us do not like to be told what to do. The objective of stopping the bad habit becomes a battle between you and your friend or loved one. This causes resentment between you. When we personally decide that we need to quit a bad habit, our success rate goes up. The decision to make healthy choices has to come from within us, not outside of us. It isn't an easy task to lose weight and have a lifestyle of healthy choices. This does not mean that friends and families should not encourage these changes. Positive reinforcements can be very helpful in this journey.

Couples Influence Each Other's Bad and Good Habits

Over the years during my weight loss patient consultations, if the patient has a significant other, it is usually easier to be on a diet or a healthy program if both parties are focused on similar goals. Before discussing how relationships and friendships can positively help individuals improve their health and accomplish weight loss, I think it important to say that we need be wary of potential negative consequences that can result from our close relationships.

For years I have watched the process when both parties in a relationship are taking part in the same bad habit such as smoking or drinking alcohol in excess. If both parties have the same unhealthy habit, it often reinforces their bad behaviors. I personally was in a relationship in which my partner often liked to have one or two glasses of wine every night. The wine was a very important part of her life. She had great knowledge of the different wines and had been around the world sampling and drinking these great wines. Wine had not been that important to me in my life. Over the years I may have at the most one alcoholic drink a week. However, because I was in a relationship and trying to blend our lives, I too began to have a glass of wine every night with my partner, and before long I was drinking one or two glasses at night. I was falling into the same trap I had been warning my patients about for years. Fortunately, I soon realized what was happening and knew I had to quit drinking altogether to stay off that slippery slope.

We must be aware that our friends or intimate partners can unknowingly sabotage us on our quest to improve our health. If your friends don't want to exercise, stop drinking alcohol, or simply don't want to address their health issues, they may consciously or unconsciously try to thwart your personal efforts to improve your own health. Your unhealthy friend or significant other might not want you to get healthier because they don't want to lose their drinking buddy or the person they meet at the donut shop. Finally, your less healthy sidekick might unconsciously not want you to get healthier because they don't want to look in the mirror and admit how unhealthy their own lifestyle has been. And the truth is that it's much simpler to sit on the couch and hangout with your good friend or loved one than to get up and go for a long walk.

The positive approach to an improved health with your partner or friend is to choose to work together to create healthy choices. As easy as it was to get unhealthy together, it can be just as easy to become healthy together, especially if you work as a team. It can be as simple as getting up early in the morning and meeting your best friend for a long walk. Many of us don't want to take on our health improvement by ourselves, but when your significant other or good friend is right there with you, it seems so much easier to accomplish. An additional benefit of being on this healthy path together is often an improved relationship. Working together on a positive goal normally only builds a stronger bond.

The bottom line is that it is much easier to eat better and exercise more if you are with someone who wants to support you, and best of all, try to emulate you and follow along on the same healthy course. However, you should not hold the health train back because your partner is not ready. When your energy is moving forward to weight loss and a healthier living, then you should just jump on that train and go and hope your friend will at some point in the future get on board with you.

A well written book called *Love Me Slender: How Smart Couples Team Up to Lose Weight* by Thomas Bradbury, PhD., and Benjamin Karney, PhD, addresses this issue of the best way couples can work together to lose weight and get healthier. The authors explain how couples are already working on other long-term projects together like raising kids, paying monthly bills, and caring for aging parents. So why not work on their weight and health together? Teaming up can often make major projects much easier to accomplish.

This book quotes several studies that showed partners in a relationship are frequently highly similar as far as their health. They often have the same physical dimensions. If one partner is becoming overweight, it is common for their partner to be overweight, too. Likewise, if one partner feels they need to lose weight, their partner may also want to lose weight. As long as this doesn't become an unfortunate competition as both partners work to attain the same goal, they usually give each other support to help increase the odds of success.

Mutual support considerably increases the odds of a being successful with your goal of weight loss. Not having mutual support can become obvious when your partner decides to pick up a dozen donuts at the bakery on the way home from work or wants to stop at the Dairy Queen when you are out together doing an errand.

The good news is that studies show partners often take part in the same wellness paths. Both, for example, generally get their flu shots and Covid-19 vaccines at the same time. So if one partner is moving in the right direction in their health, often their partner will also have the same goal. I see this all the time in my neighborhood. Whenever I am off on my bike at the crack of dawn, I see more couples walking, cycling, and running together than I see individuals exercising by themselves.

Unfortunately, the authors of *Love Me Slender* point out that just as couples follow each other to improve their health, both members of a pair also tend to move together in the opposite direction of ill health. One study showed that when a husband becomes obese the chance of his wife becoming obese is 44 %. When the wife becomes obese the risk of the husband also becoming obese is 37%.[54]

So knowing this the authors of *Love Me Slender* point to three principles couples should follow to positively influence themselves to healthy living and weight loss. The principles are:

○ The Principle of Mutual Influence

○ The Principle of Mutual Understanding

○ The Principle of Long-Term Commitment

Having a Principle of Mutual Influence

Our influence on our partner is the defining feature of any intimate relationship. This influence is powerful, irreplaceable, and inevitable.

Having a Principle of Mutual Understanding

Wanting to help is great but knowing how is crucial. Our partner holds up the mirror about who we really are. For partners to be successful they need to be able to point out your mirror in a mutual understanding way and to show the partner they understand them not that they simple have heard them.

Having a Principle of Long-Term Commitment

To make a goal in the future we often have to make certain concessions in the present. In the battle between the needs of the present and our goals for the future commitments gives us a fighting chance. Commitment to health is really the same as a commitment to a relationship. It gives us the ability to transcend the current moment in pursuit of long-term goals.

Approaching a Partner About Healthy Choices

It can be a delicate dance initially on how and when to approach your unhealthy partner to go along with you in your quest to make healthy choices. As a family physician I have consoled many couples about this issue. The best approach is to let your friend or partner know that you are making a commitment to improve your health, and if they would like to join along that would be great, but if not, that is okay. If at any point down the road they, too, would like to improve their lifestyle, you would be happy if they joined you. If both you and your friend or partner are not at an ideal weight, and you would like to lose some pounds, having your partner eat a healthier lower-calorie diet along with you rather than having to make two separate meals, would make both your lives much easier.

One last point on this topic is that it is very important to know how your partner responds to suggestions or criticisms. For example, many people do not want to be told that they need to become healthier and lose weight. This trait is certainly not limited to the male gender but is a common theme among many of them. In fact, many will go in the opposite direction and eat more, drink more, and move less if told they need to improve their health. Finding ways to encourage and persuade your friend or significant other to go along with you gives you the best odds of being successful in improving your health and losing weight.

A Deeper Dive into Weight Loss

7

Processed Foods

What is the big deal about processed foods, and why should it be featured in a weight loss book? The reason is that since we are changing our diet to help us lose weight, we might as well change it totally—not only to help us succeed in our goal of losing weight but to make us healthier. One of the biggest problems with modern-day nutrition is that the food industry, in their quest to entice individuals to eat more of their products and to keep them from spoiling, puts too many additives in our food. And adding more sugars and fats, which we all love, makes us want to buy more varieties of food and eat them on a regular basis. This has resulted in two major problems:

1. We are now eating more calorically dense foods, which causes us to gain weight.

2. Just as important, and in some ways even more important, is that these additives and changes in the processing of food increase the risk for chronic disease.

To understand why we need to limit processed foods, let's first define what they are. There are three major categories of processed foods.

- o **Unprocessed or minimally processed foods:** In general, these are the raw foods that we take directly from their natural environment, such as trees, the ground, or the ocean. Examples are vegetables, grains, legumes, fruits, nuts, meats, seafood, herbs, spices, garlic, eggs, and milk.

- o **Processed foods:** In this category of foods we add certain ingredients to the raw agricultural products such as oil, sugar or salt to foods and then package them. Some examples are canned beans and cheese. These foods have been altered, but not in a way that's detrimental to health. They are convenient and help you build nutritious meals.

- o **Ultra-processed foods:**[55] These foods go through multiple processing and contain many additives. The raw agricultural commodities may be washed, cleaned or chopped and heated, cooked, pasteurized, dehydrated, frozen, and mixed with additives such as preservatives, flavors, and other food nutrients that have been approved for food products and then sealed in metal, glass, paper, or plastic containers. Examples are soft drinks, cereals, hotdogs, potato chips, candy, and lovely chicken nuggets. Several surveys assessing individual food intake, household food expenses, or supermarket sales have suggested that ultra-processed food products contribute to between 25% and 50% of total daily energy intake. Ultra-processed foods are designed to create highly profitable (low-cost ingredients with a long shelf-life), convenient (ready-to-consume), hyper-palatable products.

Now let's look at some of the studies showing potential negative effects that may be caused by processed foods.

A paper published in *Nutrients* reviewed 43 previous studies. In 37 of those reviewed it found dietary UPF (Ultra-Processed Foods) exposure was associated with at least one adverse health outcome. Among adults, these included overweight, obesity, and cardio-metabolic risks; cancer, type-2 diabetes and cardiovascular diseases; irritable bowel syndrome, depression and all-cause mortality. Among children and adolescents, these included cardio-metabolic risks and asthma. Interestingly, **no study reported an association between UPF and beneficial health outcomes.**[56]

In another huge study in France a total of 110,260 adult participants (≥18 years old, mean baseline age = 43.1 [SD 14.6] years; 78.2% women) from the French prospective population-based NutriNet-Santé cohort (2009–2019) were included. Dietary intakes were collected at baseline using repeated and validated 24-hour dietary records linked to a food composition database that included >3,500 different food items, each categorized according to their degree of processing. Associations between the proportion of UPF in the diet and BMI change during follow-up were assessed using linear mixed models. Conclusion: In this large observational prospective study, higher consumption of UPF was associated with gain in BMI and higher risks of overweight and obesity.[57]

In summary, if you are serious about losing weight and decreasing your risk of future diseases such as cancer and cardiovascular disease, the less ultra-processed foods (UPF) you eat, the better. We can do our best to be purists and try to avoid UPFs altogether. In our society unless you eat only organic foods, and all your meals are made at home, this may be difficult. However, the closer you can get to that purified state, the healthier you will be, and the easier it may be to lose weight.

8

Intermittent Fasting and Other Trendy Diets

There is always a new diet craze. Everyone wants to jump on the bandwagon with the newest diet that is guaranteed to help a person lose weight. As I said earlier in this book, if one has been out of control in what they eat and not exercising on a regular basis, any program is often at least temporarily a good program. That is why so many new fad diets seem to work. If we follow the guidelines of a new diet or exercise, we are at least doing something rather than not doing anything to address our weight. Let's look at two of the more popular diets and discuss the pros and cons of each.

Intermittent Fasting

At the time of the writing of this book, one of the more popular diets for weight loss is Intermittent Fasting. The premise of how this diet works is that if you are not eating carbs, your carb storage dries up and therefore you must burn up fats for energy. Small studies have been mixed as to efficacy of utilizing intermittent fasting to lose weight.[58]

There are basically two types of Intermittent Fasting: one is **alternative day fasting** and the other is **time-restricted fasting**. In **alternative day fasting** it may consist of a 24-hour fast followed by a 24-hour eating period that can be done several times a week. One type of **alternate day fasting** is the 5:2 diet. With this diet there are 2 fast days mixed in with 5 nonrestrictive days. Some 5:2 diets aren't a complete fast on the 2 "fasting" days but are a very restrictive caloric diet. Mosely in his book *"The 5/2 Diet"* has men eating only 600 calories and women eating only 500 calories on those 2 days. With the **time-restricted fasting**, an individual eats meals only during a specific time frame, from 4 hours (example: 2 p.m. to 6 p.m.) up to 8 hours (example: 11 a.m. to 7 p.m.), and the rest of the time a person does not eat. The difference between a purely caloric-restricted diet and Intermittent Fasting is that during the feeding phase of Intermittent Fasting (IF) there is no calorie restriction.

What are the Pros and Cons of an Intermittent Fasting diet?

Pros:

○ There are no food restrictions on non-fasting days.

○ It's easy to follow.

○ One does not have to count calories unless their specific diet allows 600 calories for men and 500 calories for women on the fasting days.

Cons:

○ It is not recommended for individuals under the age of 18, those that could potentially become pregnant, or are breastfeeding.

○ One must be reminded to drink fluids during the fasting phase. Many of us equate food and drink, and when we are not eating, we often do not drink enough.

○ Fasting can be stressful on the body so there is a concern of increased cortisol production, which we learned in the medication chapter, can lead to weight gain.

○ Overeating and binge eating are two potential side effects of intermittent fasting. Therefore intermittent fasting is not a diet for an individual with a history of an eating disorder.

○ Fatigue is a common problem on the fasting days. This can lead to decreased physical activity, which is not what you want to do when you are trying to lose weight.

○ There has been a concern that the swings in eating may affect a person's mood.[59]

Additional negative aspects of Intermittent Fasting

1. "Hangry" (One can become irritable and bad tempered when they are hungry and haven't eaten for a prolonged time.)

2. Brain fog

3. Developing food obsessions about when you can eat

4. Hypoglycemia

5. Alopecia (hair loss)

6. Changes in the menstrual cycle

7. Constipation

8. Possibility of unhealthy dietary choices during non-fasting time

   ○ Concern about developing a binge-eating disorder (BED)

9. Sleep disturbances

   ○ Decrease in REM sleep

10. Sustainability is unlikely or not advised

One of the proposed benefits of intermittent fasting that was noted in the media was that this diet increased longevity. According to the National Institute of Aging, studies of rodents, revealed that when mice are put on a program that severely restrict diets, many show an expansion of lifespan and decreased serious diseases, especially cancer. We should note that this was a rodent study, and no long-term human studies have been done to prove or disprove the efficacy of fasting.

While the practice of intermittent fasting is not new, much of the research investigating the benefits of this routine of eating is relatively recent. For that reason, it is hard to tell if the benefits are long-lasting. Researchers often comment that long-term studies are needed to determine if the eating plan is even safe to follow for more than several months. For now if you decide to do Intermittent Fasting please consider a discussion with your health care provider because of the safety issues associated with it.

The Keto Diet

Another very popular kind of diet is the ketogenic diet. The focus is to decrease carbohydrate intake. When there are no carbs to break down for energy the body must then metabolize fats for energy. The term "ketogenic diet" generally refers to a diet that is very low in carbohydrate, modest in protein, and high in fat. This combination of macronutrients can induce ketosis. Ketosis occurs when the body produces ketone bodies to supply energy for the body when it does not have enough glucose to perform that job. If you are in a ketotic state those ketones will spill over into the urine. Therefore, urinary ketone levels are often used as an indicator of dietary adherence. This is why many who are committed to this diet will test their urine for ketones to make sure they are complying with the diet.

It is important to note that high-fat, low-carbohydrate ketogenic diets (KDs) are not new. This type of diet was first developed in the 1920s to treat pediatric refractory seizure disorders. In recent years the use of what we call "KDs" has experienced a revival to include the treatment of adulthood epilepsies as well as conditions ranging from autism to chronic pain and cancer.[60]

A Ketogenic Diet Summary

○ A typical diet contains 48% carbohydrates, 32% fat, and 17% protein. Whereas most ketogenic diets start with carbohydrate restriction of less than 10% of energy intake for about 2 months before starting a slow reintroduction.

○ Weight loss peaks at about 5 months; then weight is slowly regained.

○ Individuals that are on ketogenic diets have a tendency to eat less food. This appears to be related to a decreased appetite that is often seen in the Keto diet with its composition of higher fat and protein compared to a more typical diet containing a higher carbohydrate content.

○ Observational data suggest long-term low carbohydrate intake might be associated with increased mortality.[61]

There are several concerns I have with the ketogenic diets. Extreme carbohydrate restriction can profoundly affect diet quality. Very-low-carbohydrate diets may lack vitamins, minerals, fiber, and phytochemicals found in fruits, vegetables, and whole grains. Low-carbohydrate diets are often low in thiamin, folate, vitamin A, vitamin E, vitamin B6, calcium, magnesium, iron, and potassium.[62]

Ketogenic diets are typically low in fiber, which is needed not only for healthful intestinal function but also for microbial production of beneficial colonic short-chain fatty acids, which enhance nutrient absorption, stimulate the release of satiety hormones, improve immune function, and has anti-inflammatory and anti-carcinogenic effects. Inadequate intake of these microbiota-accessible carbohydrates found in plant cell walls also increases gut permeability.[63]

Intake of other protective dietary components normally found in many fruits and vegetables appear to be significantly lacking in a Keto diet. Examples are phytochemicals like flavanones and anthocyanins, which are antioxidants that help prevent chronic diseases such as cancers.

Most individuals who go all in with a low-carb ketogenic diet are so excited initially because they often observe a sudden rapid weight loss. Most people think it is due to loss of fat, but in reality the early rapid weight loss is most likely due to a loss of fat-free mass, which includes body water, glycogen, protein, and contents of the gastrointestinal tract.[64] The body is designed to use glucose for fuel, and when it is taken away because of the low carb diet, the body immediately goes for stored glucose, which is called glycogen. Glycogen is in the liver and muscles. It is stored glucose that is held together by simple water bonds. When the body breaks down the glycogen molecules to access the glucose, water is released and is eventually eliminated through the kidneys. So that initial weight loss is not a loss in fat. It is only a loss in water from the glycogen bonds.

An increased level of inflammation with a ketogenic diet is also a concern. In the 2021 metabolic ward trial by Hall et al. comparing the effects of an animal-based ketogenic diet and a plant-based, low-fat diet, the inflammatory maker for inflammation called the high-sensitivity C-reactive protein was substantially higher while on the ketogenic diet as compared to the plant-based diet (2.1 vs. 1.2 mg/L; $p = 0.003$).[65]

One last comment on the Keto diet is the prevailing concern that it may contribute to developing Non-Alcoholic Fatty Liver Disease (NAFLD). In epidemiological studies, diets high in saturated fat, *trans* fat, simple sugars, and animal protein (especially from red and processed meat) and low in dietary fiber and omega-3 fatty acids are thought to contribute to NAFLD. In the Rotterdam Study, those consuming the most animal protein were 54% more likely to have NAFLD than those consuming the least (OR 1.54, 95% CI, 1.20–1.98). Dietary components associated with reduced NAFLD risk include whole grains, nuts and seeds, monounsaturated fats, omega-3 fatty acids, vegetable protein, prebiotic fiber, probiotics, resveratrol, coffee, taurine, and choline.[66]

Both these diets along with many other diets seem to work at first but they don't seem to have staying power. Less than 20% of people that lose weight are able to maintain that weight loss.[67] A common scenario I have witnessed over the years has been if I meet someone who I haven't seen for a while and they look great because they have lost a significant amount of weight. When you ask them how they were able to lose their excess weight, more often than not they will tell you they did it by following one of the new fad diets. Unfortunately, the next time you see them, they often have gained back the weight they lost, and many times they gained back more weight they originally lost. They will tell you they just could not maintain that crazy diet, and it did not fit into their lifestyle. They sometimes say that if only they had lost their weight by a reasonably healthy approach, they could still be absent those pounds.

9

Emotional States and Weight Gain

The purpose of this chapter is to help people understand how a person's emotional state can have a major influence on their weight and overall health. Weight gain and the inability to lose weight may be more than overeating or not exercising enough. I have yet to see a patient who is overweight and struggling to trim down who does not have at least one emotional overlay that either influenced their weight gain or somehow has been sabotaging their ability to lose weight. The sooner the person recognizes this fact and addresses these issues, the easier it will be to lose those unwanted pounds.

It does not take a rocket scientist to realize that our emotional state can affect how we eat. We can have all the best intentions in the world at the beginning of the week to eat only certain foods and not overeat. Then, out of nowhere, we are suddenly thrown a curve ball. We may have an out-of-control teenager in our home or the family pet is gravely ill and we must do everything we can to save its life. If these stressful situations coincide, we find ourselves overeating and also selecting foods we were doing our best to avoid. This is "emotional eating." We define it as eating in response to emotional stress or triggers in our lives instead of relying on physical cues to indicate it's time to satisfy our hunger.

People in this state eat mindlessly without awareness of the reasons for overeating or regard for our loss of discipline. This behavior is often a result of psychological distress from trauma, depression, and anxiety caused by isolation and loneliness.[68] People who become "emotional eaters" often have food obsessions. They obsess about when their next meal will be and may spend excessive amounts of money on food. While overeating is not a diagnosable condition, if left untreated or unchecked, the behavior can potentially lead to other more serious eating disorders such as Bulimia Nervosa and Binge Eating Disorder (BED).[69]

It has long been felt that excessive stress, often caused by previous trauma, is a major cause of weight gain. Studies have shown that PTSD (Post-Traumatic Stress Syndrome) participants exhibited greater emotional eating than control participants, and the degree of emotional eating increased with higher PTSD symptom severity. The obvious result of abnormal overeating is weight gain.[70]

Additional Studies of the Association of Stressful Events and Weight Gain

1. Considerable evidence from both population-based and clinical studies indicates a significant and positive association of high stressful events with both substance addiction and weight gain.[71]

2. Stressful events such as job strain, unemployment, family caregiving, marital conflicts, and chronic adversity including poverty are associated with weight gain. [72]

Benefits of Meditation to Help to Relieve Stress

If you are dealing with stressors that are affecting how you eat, there are some simple techniques you can do that may help you. One technique is learning to meditate. There are several good apps out there that can help you get started. The one I recommend the most is Headspace. It guides you through a very simple meditation that lasts only about ten minutes. A practice of a daily meditation (and it can be only ten minutes) has been shown to decrease stress and decrease cortisol levels.[73]

Another simple technique is to learn a breathing method to help you when you start to be stressed. It is important to note that the farther along a person is in becoming acutely stressed, the more difficult it is to help the individual to relax. The easy breathing technique I advise is the 4-6-8 method. You begin by slowly counting in your head to 4 as you take in a slow deep breath. Then hold your breath for a count of 6 and then exhale for a slow 8 count. Repeat this several times when you are starting to feel stressed. You may be amazed how this simple little technique can help calm you down. Finally, remember that the earlier you recognize you are feeling stressed-out, the easier it is to stop it and prevent abnormal eating patterns.

What else can we do about emotional eating? The common triggers are trauma, stressors in our family, relationship issues, and occupational stress. If you are dealing with these situations and are struggling with your weight, you should consider seeking out some kind of help for your emotional problems. Help can be in the form of seeing a behavioral therapist such as a psychologist or social worker, or getting advice from your family doctor, a supportive family member, or perhaps a very supportive friend. Emotional eating is an obstacle that needs to be addressed ideally before, or at least at the same time, you spend hours trying to exercise or embark on a new diet program. Until these emotional issues are dealt with, they will continue to be a roadblock to your goal of attaining a healthy weight.

There are other mental states that can affect how we eat and how often we eat. One such mindset is called "mindless eating." This simply means we are eating without really thinking about what we are eating. Some examples of this are eating in front of the TV, eating while reading the newspaper, or eating while working on the computer. People that eat mindlessly have the tendency to overeat and may even eat food they don't like.[74] Another version of this thoughtless eating is unconsciously grabbing something to eat every time you walk by the refrigerator or the pantry. You have cheese, crackers, or chips in your mouth before you realize it. Often when this happens you weren't even hungry in the first place. The book *Mindless Eating: Why We Eat More Than We Think* by Brian Wansink describes how these hidden factors eventually lead to an increase in caloric intake over time and results in a slow and subtle weight gain.

So what do we do about this mindless eating? The simple answer is that we need to be more aware, present, and conscious when we eat. A way of doing this is through "Mindful Eating." Mindfulness in general was defined by John Kabat-Zinn, the founder in 1982 of the program for meditation practice called Mindfulness-Based Stress Reduction (MSBR defined his operational definition of mindfulness as "The awareness that arises through paying attention, on purpose, in the present moment, nonjudgmentally.") (from the YouTube video "Peel Back the Onion" made in 12/8/2016)

The following text is quoted from statements by The Center for Mindful Eating:*

> Mindful eating involves bringing one's full attention to the process of eating, including focusing on all the tastes, smells, thoughts, and feelings that arise during a meal. . . . Those who mindfully eat are more aware of their emotions and physical sensations in the moment and can work to reach a state of full attention to food, such as their decisions around food, hunger cues, and satiety.

---

* The Center for Mindful Eating (TCME) is a member-supported, nonprofit international organization. Our mission is to help people achieve a balanced, healthy, respectful, and joyful relationship with food and eating. TCME provides resources for educating professionals, institutions, and individuals in the principles and practices of mindful eating. (thecenterformindfuleating.org)

The center goes on to further define someone who eats mindfully as:

> ... one who acknowledges that there is no right or wrong way to eat but varying degrees of awareness surrounding the experience of food and accepts that their eating experiences are unique.

Individuals who practice mindful eating direct their attention to eating on a moment-by-moment basis and gaining awareness of how they can make choices that support health and well-being. The reality is that when we eat mindlessly, we commonly overeat. So being more conscious and aware when we eat, and how we feel when we eat, can decrease the intake portion of the eating equation.

The Importance of Having a Sense of Purpose in Life to Achieve Weight Loss and Healthy Behaviors

Those individuals that are more susceptible to emotional eating are often those who have a low self-esteem, lack some type of spiritual fulfillment, and have lost their sense of purpose. This was shown in a study of a group of college women who had feelings of low spiritual well-being and expressed they lacked a sense of purpose. They were found to have a much higher level of emotional overeating than controls.[75]

Accumulating evidence shows that a higher sense of purpose in life is associated with lower risk of chronic conditions and premature mortality. A study that followed 13,770 adults over eight years showed those in the top versus the lowest quartile of those who feel they have a purpose in life had 24% lower likelihood of becoming physically inactive, 33% lower likelihood of developing sleep problems, and 22% lower likelihood of developing unhealthy body mass index (BMI). These findings remained evident even after further adjusting for baseline health status and depression. These results suggest that a sense of purpose in life might emerge as a valuable target to consider for interventions aimed at helping adults maintain healthy behaviors.[76] The bottom line is that if you find yourself wandering around in life feeling you have little purpose, your ability to lose weight becomes more difficult. Working with your health provider, a professional counselor, spiritual guide, close friends, or family about finding your sense of life's purpose, and having direction toward that purpose may pay back big dividends in the long run in your pursuit of better health.

In this chapter we learned how emotions and mindsets can affect a person's weight. I would be remiss if I didn't discuss the importance of motivation in a person's ability to lose weight. One of the biggest advantages of working at Canyon Ranch is the high level of motivation my patients have when they come to see me. When I was in private practice before I came to Canyon Ranch, I saw people that were overweight and out of control of their health. I would spend most of the office visit trying to motivate the patient to make lifestyle changes to improve their health and prevent chronic disease. Sadly, most of those patient's concerns were only about their immediate health issues. They did not want to be bothered about the potential of future health problems. I always had to work very hard to try to motivate them to make changes in their life to prevent future disease. Here at Canyon Ranch, I am blessed that the majority of my patients are already well-motivated to make healthy changes in their life to improve their overall health.

With this viewpoint, half the battle is already won. I think the take-home here is that initially we all need a pep talk before we embark on a weight loss program, and the main pep talk must come from within ourselves. We need to be totally convinced this is the right thing to do and totally committed to it. Your path to weight loss will be much easier if you have a positive mindset and are well-motivated to take on this task.

The Future and Next Steps

10

Maintaining Weight Loss

So now that you have lost weight, how can you keep that weight off? This is always the big overriding question. The numbers are not in your favor. Depending on what you read, only 15 to 20% of people who have lost a significant amount of weight are able to keep it off. The typical weight-loss pattern seen in most studies, whether it's through changes in lifestyle, pharmacologic treatments, or surgical procedures for obesity, results in a varying degree of weight loss over the first 6 to 9 months. This is followed by a plateau period with a subsequent period of weight regain. Weight loss generally occurs over a limited period of time, whereas maintenance of reduced weight requires a lifetime of diligent attention.[77]

Over my 40 years of practicing medicine I have seen many patients who were able to lose weight either through individual effort or a structured weight loss program. Over the years, whenever I saw patients who had lost a significant amount of weight, I would praise them and tell them how happy I was about their ability to lose that weight. I relayed to them that with their weight loss the potential to have a long-term healthy life was exponentially increased. I would point out all the positive physiological changes that may have already occurred or can come about in the future because they are less heavy, such as an improved blood pressure and blood sugar.

What was so discouraging to me, and especially to the patients themselves, was that over time many of them who had been so excited to come in to see me to show off their weight loss would avoid seeing me in further follow-up visits. The reason they did not come back to visit me was that they had gained back the weight they had worked so hard to lose. Often they gained back more weight than what they originally lost. They were not scheduling follow-up visits with me because of their self-imposed shame from gaining back all that weight. This was so frustrating. When I did finally see them, I would tell them that losing weight is much like quitting smoking. It is not uncommon for someone to attempt to quit smoking once, twice, and even three times before they actually quit. I would tell them they needed to attempt to lose that weight again. If they were successful in losing a lot of pounds once, they have the knowledge and capability to do it again.

So what happened? After hours of sacrifice and effort people lost all this weight, but then up to 85% of them ended up slipping and falling and before long were right back to where they started. Instead of focusing on who and why people failed, let's first look at the 15% of individuals who have been successful and see if we can learn from them their secrets of achievement.

By far the largest ongoing study looking at individuals with successful "long-term" weight-loss, is the National Weight Loss Registry. This study was established in 1994 by Rena Wing, Ph.D. from Brown Medical School, and James O. Hill, Ph.D. from the University of Colorado. It is the largest prospective investigation of long-term successful weight loss maintenance. The NWCR has been tracking over 10,000 individuals over the age of 18 who have lost significant amounts of weight and kept it off for long periods of time. To be in the study you must have lost a minimum of 30 pounds (some people have lost up to 300 pounds) and were able to keep that weight off for a minimum of one year. In this group the average length of time they have been able to maintain their weight loss is 5.5 years, and their average weight loss is 66 pounds. In other words, these are the true winners of weight loss.

So what are the key points that have come from this study?

1. 45% of registry participants lost the weight on their own, and the other 55% lost weight with the help of some type of program. *Therefore, usage of an outside source to help you lose weight seems to have some benefit.*

2. 98% of Registry participants report that they modified their food intake in some way to lose weight. *This indicates the majority of people prior to starting their weight program more than likely had poor dietary habits.*

3. 94% of the participants increased their physical activity, with walking the most frequently reported form of activity. *This confirms that if we are couch potatoes, we need to get moving and increase our physical activity and continue it to maintain our weight loss.*

4. Most members of this group report maintaining a low calorie, low fat diet.

5. Additional points of interest about this group:

    ○ 78% ate breakfast every day.
    ○ 75% weigh themselves at least once a week.
    ○ 62% watch less than 10 hours of TV per week.
    ○ 90% exercise, on average, 1 hour per day.

In addition to what we have learned from the NWCR group, many other studies have looked at the issue of maintaining weight loss. One such study showed that in order to maintain weight loss we must conserve our lean mass (our muscles) as we lose weight. This is a major key in sustaining weight loss, especially as we get older. We may be able to lose weight through diet and aerobic exercise, but in order to keep that weight off we need the engine to continue to burn up those calories. If in the process of losing weight a person loses muscle mass, they won't be able to burn up enough calories to keep that weight off. So we must preserve our muscles after we lose weight, and in some cases must increase our muscle mass as we embark on a diet-restricted program.[78]

Other studies performed to analyze those individuals who were successful in keeping their weight off showed some interesting findings:[79]

1. Individuals that continued to self-monitor their weight and their eating were more likely to be successful in maintaining their new weight. *I hear all the time from my patients that they did not want to get on the scales because it was too emotional for them. The fact is if you want to be successful at keeping your weight off, you need to consistently check in to see how you are doing.*

2. Individuals who increased their exercise program and maintained that higher level of exercise were more likely to keep their weight off.

3. Eating behaviors such as portion control, cutting out unhealthy foods, and reducing energy intake, were found to be positively predictive of weight loss maintenance.

4. Strong evidence supported the facts that eating out and the use of meal replacements were non-significant in predicting weight loss maintenance. *So if you want to go out for dinner **occasionally**, it's okay!*

5. At the product level, an increase in fruit and vegetable consumption and a reduction in sugar-sweetened beverages were positively predictive of weight loss maintenance.

6. Decrease fat intake was found to be positively predictive of weight loss maintenance.

   Be careful with this one. Yes, less fat is helpful in both weight loss and maintaining that weight loss, but it doesn't mean grabbing up all those low-fat processed foods that end up replacing their zero-fat food with a boatload of carbs. It means you should consume less animal and dairy fat.

7. Self-efficacy for exercise and self-efficacy for weight management were strongly supported to be positively predictive of weight loss maintenance.

   (Self-efficacy refers to an individual's belief in their capacity to execute behaviors necessary to produce specific performance attainments.)

8. Having high self-esteem about yourself was found to be positively predictive of weight loss maintenance.

   In other words, if you like yourself, you will have a higher likelihood of being successful.

9. Family discouragement of healthy eating and regular exercise were measured and were reported to be negatively predictive of weight loss maintenance.

   You need your family to rally around and support you as you keep your weight off and not discourage you.

10. Commercial weight loss programs were found NOT to be significantly predictive of weight loss maintenance.

11. The weight a person started with did not seem to influence their success rate in keeping their weight off.

    Therefore it doesn't matter what weight you are starting from; the ability to keep your weight off is the same.

Another important aspect of individuals that were successful in weight loss maintenance is close follow-up. Being accountable to someone other than ourselves seems to be beneficial.[80] In other words, you can't get away with anything when someone is looking over your shoulder! This can be done with support groups like Overeaters Anonymous or being followed by a health coach. At Canyon Ranch we also have a health coach who stays in contact with our patients after they leave the ranch. This has been very successful. It's that constant check-in with a health coach that keeps our patients on track with their weight loss. I am not saying everyone needs someone hovering over them to stay on their diet and exercise program, but for a significant number of individuals, it seems to be a very important part of those that are successful in weight maintenance.

If you don't want to work with other humans to get support, there are plenty of Apps now that seem to hover over us to keep us on track. An example is the Apple 10,000 steps. I cannot tell you how many times patients, staff, and friends want to point out to me how many steps they have accomplished that day. It's not really a support system but sets up an emotional check-in that often keeps a person on track and reminds them daily that this is a lifelong commitment to a healthy life.

So what is the science behind this difficulty in maintaining weight loss? It has been shown that individuals become both hypometabolic (have a slower metabolism) and hyperphagic (have increased appetite) after they lose at least 10% of their body weight. Some of this may be explained by a reduction of leptin (the hormone that suppresses our appetite) that has been noted with weight loss. Another important source of this hypometabolic state is related to improved skeletal muscle efficiency. The decline in non-resting energy expenditure (NREE) is due mainly to an approximate 20 percent increase in skeletal muscle chemo-mechanical contractile efficiency during low levels of energy expenditure. This "hypometabolism" persists in individuals for a long period of time.[81] As a result, when we become conditioned to our workouts, we don't spend as much energy with each exercise as we did when we began our exercise program. This makes total sense when you compare how you felt during your workout the first time you started to train compared to how you felt about working out after a few weeks of training. As you become more conditioned, you burn up less calories with that same physical activity.

Another scientific basis for the difficulty in maintaining weight loss is that loss of weight provokes declines in sympathetic nervous system activity and increases in parasympathetic nervous system activity. These changes combine to reduce both Resting Energy Expenditure (REE) and Non-Resting Energy Expenditure (NREE).[82] Decreased catecholamine excretion also inhibits the release of bioactive thyroid hormones. All this helps to explain why it can be an uphill battle to maintain our weight loss.

By utilizing the scientific studies we discussed, the following list is a summary of suggestions on how to keep that weight off.

1. All of us can modify our diet to make it healthier. What makes a diet healthy? Of course, that can be a whole book in itself. Some simple rules of a healthy diet are:

   ○ A person needs to eat at least 3 to 5 servings of fruits and vegetables a day. (The nutritionists at Canyon Ranch would like you to eat 5 to 9 servings, but get started with a bare minimum of 3, and then work your way up.) Make the meal plate look colorful with various colors of fruits and vegetables. This increases the number of vitamins, minerals, and antioxidants a person will ingest.

   ○ Limit red meat.

   ○ Eat more omega 3 foods such as fish (non-predatory) and ground flax seed, and so forth.

- ○ Be wary of overeating. Remember what a portion size is. (One portion equals about the size of a small fist.)

- ○ Be sure it is a sustainable diet that is not so restrictive that it can only be maintained for a short period of time.

2. Start or continue an exercise program to be at least 3 days a week but preferably 5 days a week. Be prepared to up your exercise program if it seems like every time you finish your exercise you feel you could easily go longer. Remember that you won't burn up as many calories as you become conditioned.

3. Eat breakfast. Not an absolute must-have, but remember that 78% of the successful participants in the NWR ate breakfast.

4. Have routine check-ins to be sure you are on track. Examples are obtaining daily or weekly weights.

5. Limit TV and computer (non-work related) exposure.

6. Reduce sugar-sweetened beverages and artificially sweetened beverages (to be discussed more in the next chapter).

7. Limit highly processed foods.

8. Believe in yourself, and believe that you can do this.

9. Surround yourself with people that will give you positive reinforcement on your quest to maintain a healthy weight.

11

Gut Microbiome and Artificial Sweeteners

Microbiome

The gut microbiome is the totality of a person's microorganisms, bacteria, viruses, protozoa, and fungi, and their collective genetic material in the gastrointestinal tract. The make-up of an individual's microbiome is generally determined by their third or fourth year of life. This is driven by many factors, including breast-feeding, a person's age, sex, and the food they eat. These microorganisms have a major influence on our health in many different venues. They can affect our metabolism, immune system, neuroendocrine responses, nutrient and mineral absorption, synthesis of enzymes, vitamins, and amino acids, and production of short-chain fatty acids (SCFAs).[83]

With the multiple influences the gut microbiome has on the body, it is not a surprise that scientific studies have also shown that the gut microbiome can affect a person's weight. One of the first landmark studies reported on this topic was an article released in 2015 that showed that the ratio of two specific bacterial phyla (a category in the scientific classification of living things)* in the gut, Firmicutes and Bacteroides, influenced whether someone was overweight or not. The study showed that the higher the ratio of the quantity Firmicutes

---

* As I describe the bacteria in the gut, it may be helpful to explain the scientific hierarchy of the classification of organisms. Most of us had to learn this in high school biology class, but I am sure the majority of us have forgotten it:
Domain>Kingdom>Phylum>Class>Order>Family>Genus>Species

bacteria to Bactroides bacteria, the greater were the odds that a person was overweight.[84]

The level of the diversity of the bacteria in the gut appears to be another influence on our weight. It has been shown that there was a negative correlation between a person's body mass index and micro-biota diversity. In other words the more diverse the bacteria are in the gut, the better we are in terms of overall health and in managing our weight.

So we know it's a good thing to have a lot of different types of bacteria in the gut (improved gut bacteria diversity), but how do we know that they are the best kinds of bacteria to improve our health? A positive indicator that a person has a good gut microbiome is if it produces a significant amount of short chain fatty acids (SCFAs). The SCFAs are acetate, propionate, and butyrate. SCFAs are produced by colonic fermentation involving anaerobic breakdown of dietary fiber and protein (Baothman, et al., 2016; Zhang et al., 2018). They are essentially the waste products produced by the gut microbes. The beneficial effects of SCFAs are numerous. They are associated with improved insulin sensitivity and glucose balance and are instrumental in strengthening the intestinal wall. They have been shown to reduce inflammation and have a positive influence on lipid (fat) metabolism. All these affects can have an impact on a person's weight.

One of the ways that SCFAs can operate is by acting on free fatty acid receptor 2 to stimulate the release of the hormone peptide YY (PYY). This hormone is released from cells in the small intestines and colon, and its major function is to reduce a person's appetite; (Brooks et al., 2016.) SCFAs also act as signaling molecules to activate at least two G-protein coupled receptors, Gpr41 and Gpr43, that promote down-stream secretion of leptin and peptide YY (PYY); both of these are appetite suppressants). SCFAs have in addition been shown to increase glucagon-like peptide (GLP1)[85] This peptide has multiple effects. It increases insulin secretion, decreases glucagon release, a hormone produced in the pancreas that causes the breakdown of stored glucose, called glycogen, into simple glucose, and it decreases stomach emptying, which will suppress appetite. Some of the new diabetic medications that are being advertised on the TV stations are GLP-1 agonists, which stimulate the GLP-1 receptors. A few of these drugs are Ozempic, Trulicity, and Rybelsus. More of the importance of this particular peptide will be discussed later in this chapter under the section about artificial sweeteners.

It is interesting to note that our diet as well as the actual makeup of a person's gut microbiome can influence the production of short chain fatty acids. The typical Western diet of high fat, high simple carbohydrates, and low fiber decreases the production of short chain fatty acids (SCFA).

We have learned that increased bacterial diversity and high production of SCFAs appears to be a good thing in improving a person's health and promoting weight loss, but what about the specific bacteria that are found in the gut. Are there some bacteria that are more beneficial than others? Over the years medicine has only focused on the disease-causing bacteria that live in the gut. Examples are salmonella, v. cholera, and typhoid. This is important if a person is sick with a fever and diarrhea, and these bacteria are the source of that illness. When this is the case, those pathogenic bacteria need to be diagnosed and eliminated. Now we are learning that we not only need to recognize pathogenic bacteria and rid ourselves of them, but we need to look for other bacteria to determine if we have "good" bacteria in our gut to help improve our health.

One such "good" bacteria is *Akkermancia. Muciniphila.* These particular bacteria have been shown to have protective effects against gut permeability and endotoxemia (toxins in your blood caused by pathogenic gram-negative bacteria; the best example is the E. coli infections that cause serious food poisoning), and it helps to reinforce the immune system and to improve glucose homeostasis. Thus individuals with higher amounts of *A. muciniphila* have a better status of health (Dao et al., 2016). Such successful studies suggest that *A. muciniphila* could find use as a next generation probiotic to combat prediabetes.[86]

I would be remiss if I didn't discuss the newer ratio of bacteria in the gut associated with health and weight loss. It is within the gram-negative Bacteroidetes phylum. It is the ratio of bacterial strains from the genus Bacteroides to genus *Prevotella.* The genus *Prevotella* produces enzymes that degrade plant fiber. The ratio of *Bacteroides/Prevotella* increases by a factor of 10 when a plant-based diet is replaced by a Western diet of high in animal protein, the nutrient choline, and saturated fat. So what does this potentially result in? Individuals with a lower versus higher gut to *Bacteroides* to *Prevotella* ratio lost significantly more weight on a calorie-restricted, high-fiber diet.[87] Once again the simplistic answer to having better gut bacteria is to eat more fruits and vegetables!

Probiotics

Should we all take **probiotics**? Even though on the surface it sounds like a good idea, the verdict is still out. Some studies demonstrate that taking a probiotic may have some promise, but most of the studies have been for a short term of less than 3 months. Because of this, we aren't sure how well probiotics work in the long-term. There are almost as many studies that show a positive effect as there are studies that show no effect. However, there are few studies that show a negative effect. There are multiple variables that may determine the efficacy of a probiotic., which is the probable reason there are so many conflicting studies.

Aspects of the person's own existing microbiome can account for different impacts of probiotics on the host. There are microbiomes that are better suited for colonization of probiotic bacteria than others.

These "permissive" microbiomes are also more prone to compositional and functional alterations in response to probiotics, and the gut epithelium of their hosts exhibits enrichment in distinct pathways compared to that of hosts with resistant microbiomes.[88] Pre-supplementation butyrate (one of the SCFAs we talked about earlier) levels are also associated with a differential effect of probiotics on the microbiome and butyrate production or metabolism. A person's diet may affect properties of probiotics, as dietary polyunsaturated fatty acids (PUFA) can modulate probiotics adhesion.

Those studies with promising outcomes with probiotics have shown their positive affects maybe a result of increasing Short Chain Fatty Acids and/or reducing quantitative lipopolysaccharide (LPS) producers, that promotes endotoxemia and organic inflammation. In addition probiotics may also inhibit fat accumulation, and insulin resistance, and regulate neuropeptides and gastrointestinal peptides.[89]

Another function is counteracting the activity of pathogenic intestinal bacteria, introduced from contaminated food and environment. Therefore, probiotics may effectively inhibit the development of pathogenic bacteria, such as *Clostridium perfringens, Campylobacter jejuni, Salmonella* Enteritidis, *Escherichia coli*, various species of *Shigella, Staphylococcus*, and *Yersinia*, thus preventing food poisoning.[90] A positive effect of probiotics on digestion processes, treatment of food allergies, candidiasis, and dental caries has been confirmed. Probiotic microorganisms such as *Lactobacillus plantarum, Lactobacillus reuteri Bifidobacterium adolescentis*, and *Bifidobacterium pseudocatenulatum* [are natural producers of B group vitamins (B1, B2, B3, B6, B8, B9, B12). They also increase the efficiency of the immunological system, enhance the absorption of vitamins and mineral compounds, and stimulate the generation of organic acids and amino acids.

Probiotic microorganisms may also be able to produce enzymes, such as esterase, lipase, and co-enzymes A, Q, NAD, and NADP, which are all involved with metabolism. Some products of probiotics' metabolism may also show antibiotic (acidophiline, bacitracin, lactacin), anti-cancerogenic, and immunosuppressive properties. Probiotics may be helpful in the treatment of inflammatory enteral conditions, including ulcerative colitis and non-specific ileitis. The etiology of those diseases is not completely understood, but it is evident that they are associated with chronic and recurrent infections or inflammations of the intestine. Clinical studies have demonstrated that probiotics can lead to the remission of ulcerative colitis, but no positive effect on Crohn's disease has been observed. Numerous studies assessed the use of probiotics in the treatment of lactose intolerance irritable bowel syndrome, and the prevention of colorectal cancer and peptic ulcers.[91]

Unfortunately an aspect of probiotics that must be known is that many of the probiotics studies are linked, funded, initiated, and endorsed by commercial entities of the probiotic industry or professional lobbying groups that are heavily associated with and funded by the same industry. While this reality by itself does not necessarily compromise the validity of such studies, there is a need to have an independent corroboration of efficacy claims through nonaffiliated research by scientific and medical entities.

Bile Acids and the Microbiome

A factor that can affect a person's microbiome, and therefore potentially affect their weight, is if they are under-producing bile acids from the liver. People that have reduced production of bile acids (an example are individuals that have cirrhosis of the liver)[92] are often associated with bacterial overgrowth and inflammation. Diet, antibiotic therapy, and disease states affect the balance of the microbiome-bile acid pool. It is clear that bile acids have a direct antimicrobial effect on gut microbes. Much of its antimicrobial effect is due to its hydrophobicity and detergent properties on bacterial membranes. Decreasing levels of bile acids in the gut favor gram-negative members of the microbiome, some of which produce potent lipopolysaccharide (LPS) and include potential pathogens.[93] The detergent activity of bile acids can disrupt bacterial cell membranes and damage DNA.

Knowing a person may have a decreased production of bile acids from certain diseases of the liver should keep that person on high alert for dysbiosis or bacterial overgrowth that may ultimately decrease a person's ability to lose weight.

Prebiotics

The World Health Organization defines prebiotics as nonviable food components that confer a health benefit on the host associated with modulation of the microbiota. In other words, prebiotics are good food for the gut bacteria but have no nutritious or caloric value to humans. Prebiotics can be used instead of probiotics or as an additional support for them.[94] Prebiotics are present in natural products, but they may also be added to food. Some examples are insulin, fructooligosaccharides, lactulose, and derivatives of galactose and β-glucans. Those substances may serve as a medium for probiotics. They stimulate their growth and contain no microorganisms.

Prebiotics are not digested by host enzymes and reach the colon in a practically unaltered form. It is there where they are fermented by saccharolytic bacteria (e.g., *Bifidobacterium* genus). The consumption of prebiotics largely affects the composition of the intestinal microbiota and its metabolic activity.

In addition to stimulating the growth and activity of beneficial bacteria in the gastrointestinal tract, prebiotics have also been shown to have many other health benefits. They increase the absorption of minerals, mostly of magnesium and calcium.

Studies on colorectal carcinoma demonstrated that the disease occurs less commonly in people who often eat vegetables and fruit. This effect is attributed mostly to the inulin and oligofructose that are in those foods. Other studies have demonstrated a reduction of the blood LDL (low-density lipoprotein) level, a stimulation of the immunological system, a maintenance of correct intestinal pH value, low caloric value, and alleviation of symptoms of peptic ulcers and vaginal mycosis. Finally the effects of inulin and oligofructose on human health are helping with lactose intolerance and dental caries treatment.[95]

Artificial and Non-Sugar Sweeteners

The usage of artificial sweeteners has gone through the roof, especially with soda drinks. In the United States, 41% of adults and 25% of children report daily consumption of artificial sweeteners.[96] There has been a big debate as to whether or not artificial or non-sugar sweeteners really help us lose weight. The big beverage companies have insinuated that they do. This is a common question on the minds of many of my patients. It seems like every time I give a presentation, at least one person in the audience will ask me what I think about artificial sweeteners. They want to know whether it is better to have a regular soft drink with sugar or a diet soft drink with artificial sweetener. That is an easy answer. Both are bad. The real question is whether an artificially sweetened drink or food is beneficial in losing weight. Let's do a deep dive and see what artificial sweeteners are and how they can affect our bodies.

Let's first use the more correct term that is used in the scientific literature for artificial sweeteners, which is **Intense Sweeteners** (IS). Next, we should know what constitutes an Intense Sweetener. Then we should ask, "How do soft-drink manufacturers claim there are zero or nearly zero calories in their drinks?

Well, they are called intense sweeteners because they are just that. These intense sweeteners are more than 30 times sweeter than sucrose, which is table sugar. Their extreme sweetness is due to higher binding affinity to sweet receptors than regular sugar. Because of this, it takes very small amounts of intense sweeteners to make the food or drink sweet. With these extremely small amounts of food substance the energy contribution is little to none. With this negligible energy contribution, it would seem logical that with the old math equation of "weight loss equals energy-in minus energy-out," this would be a very easy way to eliminate high caloric sugary foods and therefore lose weight.

Unfortunately, the scientific literature has not born this out. The first study to identify the association between artificial sweetener use and weight gain was a 1986 prospective cohort study of 78,694 women aged 50–69. This study found that artificial sweetener use was associated with increased body weight over a 1-year period.[97] Another large study was a French longitudinal study with 66,118 women that lasted over 14 years, 1369 of them developed type 2 diabetes. Importantly, there was a 68% increase in the risk of developing diabetes in those 14 years in women who consumed more than 603 mL per week of IS-containing beverages.[98]

The original intent for the use of Intense Sweeteners (IS) was to develop a substance that could combat obesity and insulin resistance and at the same time not affect the product's taste. The sad reality is that their use has been associated not only with potential weight gain, but with altered glucose homeostasis, decreased satiety signaling, increased food intake, and an altered gut microbiome. Part of the weight gain and disrupted glucose homeostasis associated with IS consumption may be explained by the alteration of levels of glucagon-like peptide-1 (GLP-1).[99] GLP-1 is a hormone, whose most notable role is in stimulating insulin secretion. It is also involved in regulating appetite and food intake by decreasing glucagon (a hormone produced in the pancreas that causes the breakdown of stored glucose, glycogen, into simple glucose) release and decreases stomach emptying, which will suppress appetite. Because of this, it may be associated with the development of type 2 diabetes.[100]

It is interesting to note that many of the new diabetic drugs stimulate this GLP-1 receptor site to improve glucose control, but unlike some of the older diabetic medications it has been shown to cause weight loss in some people. The pharmaceutical companies have recognized this and gave new names to these diabetic medications, but did not change the formula, and are now starting to market them as new weight-reducing medications. This effect may be related to the slowing of food through the stomach and small intestine that causes a decrease in appetite.

Shearer and colleagues recently demonstrated that for rats, aspartame consumption was associated with a marked impairment in both fasting blood glucose and insulin tolerance.[101] Short term stevia consumption in rats was suggested to be associated with weight gain.[102] Another group of sugar substitutes is called "sugar alcohols." They are commonly seen in sugar-free gum. Some examples are xylitol, mannitol, and sorbitol. It has been shown that they interact with, and alter the composition of, the gut microbiome, which may cause weight gain.[103]

There is mounting evidence of an association of weight gain with the ingestion of Intense Sweeteners. At this point in time the mechanism of action appears to be the interference of GLP-1 hormone and altering of the gut microbiome in such a way that it changes a person's glucose tolerance, insulin sensitivity, satiety, and possibly inflammation. Therefore, if you are downing multiple diet beverages a day because they have no calories, I would ask you to reconsider your actions and make another choice, like water.

Ways to Improve Your Microbiome

We learned earlier in this chapter that the microbiome is enormously complex, and there are specific aspects of the microbiome that when present, make it a healthier microbiome. One of the first things we look for to show that one has a healthier microbiome is an increased diversity among the microbes. We know that the more diverse the microbiome is, the lower the risk is for disease and weight gain. Another important sign that one has a healthy microbiome is its ability to produce short chain fatty acids. The advantage of producing significant amounts of SCFAs was discussed earlier in the chapter. There are ways that one can improve this diversity and increase the production of short chain fatty acids, plus additional factors that can make your microbiome healthy. The following is a list of things to do to improve the microbiome:

1. Increase fiber intake.[104] Aim for more than 40g per day, which is about double the current American average.

   ○ Eat as many types of fruits and vegetables as possible. Because of variations in fiber, the variety may be as important as the quantities. Different fibers may support distinct microbial species.

   ○ Pick high-fiber vegetables. (see the recipes at the end of this book)

2. Choose food and drinks with high levels of polyphenols.

   ○ Polyphenols are antioxidants that act as fuel for microbes. Examples are nuts, seeds, berries, olive oil, cruciferous vegetables, coffee and teas.

3. Eat plenty of fermented foods containing live microbes.

   ○ Good choices are unsweetened yogurt; kefir, which is a sour milk drink with five times as many microbes as yogurt; sauerkraut; kimchi, a Korean dish made from garlic, cabbage, and chili; and soybean-based products such as soy sauce, tempeh and natto.

4. Steer clear of artificial sweeteners.

5. Avoid processed food (see previous chapter).

6. Spend more time in the country.

    ○ People living in rural areas have better microbes than city-dwellers. Gardening and other outdoor activities are also good for your microbiome.

7. Avoid antibiotics when possible.

    ○ If you have an infection and are prescribed an antibiotic by your healthcare provider, take the antibiotic and take it until it is gone. What we are talking about here are those people who think they need an antibiotic every time they get a cold.

12

Genetics and Weight Loss

A re some of us genetically predetermined to gain weight? Is there anything we can do to prevent weight gain because of our genetic makeup? Do certain genes predispose individuals to be overweight? It's the old adage of nature versus nurture. The reality is that both nature and nurture play a part in our health and body structure (overweight, underweight or at a healthy weight). Even though this book has been focusing on the many nurture aspects that can affect our weight, it is important to know how nature (genetics) can also affect our weight.

We know that environmental factors, such as not exercising or over-eating, have been the major contributors to the recent rise in the number of people who are overweight and obese. It is also important to recognize the fact that genetic factors account for over 40–90% of the population variation in body types.[105] It is hoped that by identifying the genetic factors underlying the risk of obesity, it will contribute to our basic knowledge on how we process foods and therefore give us a better roadmap on how we approach weight loss on an individual basis.

There is a percentage of people who are born with genes that increase their risk for gaining weight. One should not have a defeatist attitude about this. By knowing your genetic makeup, it may give you an explanation as to why you have struggled with your weight over the years, and some of your friends haven't. More importantly, it may give you insights on how to reverse that weight-gaining trend and start to drop some pounds. It may illuminate to you why you have such a sweet tooth or why you can't pass up that crispy deep-fried chicken that a particular colonel makes. In other words studies have shown that there are certain lifestyles and dietary choices that can affect our health more than others based on our genetic makeup. Our genetics have even been shown to have an impact on what kind of exercise program may be better suited for us individually.

Some of the original work in looking at genes and obesity originated with the *FTO gene* region. The FTO stands for **Fat Mass and Obesity-Associated Gene**. Those individuals, with *FTO* gene *region variants*, have a higher risk for obesity. People with the *FTO variant* are much more susceptible to the weight gain from fats especially saturated fats. Fried foods are not their friend. What is also interesting is that these same groups of genetic variants are more affected by a sedentary lifestyle causing weight gain than those who do not have the variant.[106]

We in the medical and nutrition world have been talking about the ill effects associated with sugar-sweetened beverages for years. There are certain individuals who have a variant of *chromosome 9p21* that makes them especially susceptible to sugar-sweetened beverages. They have been shown to gain more weight drinking the sugar-sweetened beverages than those who do not have this chromosome.[107]

There are other genes that have a predilection for weight gain and therefore increased chronic disease risk. The APOA2 is the second most abundant apolipoprotein in HDL, the "good or happy" cholesterol. The *APOA2 variant* has an increased sensitivity to saturated fats and its presence increases the likelihood of consuming more fats. It is for this reason that people with the *APOA2 variant* need to consciously avoid saturated fats.[108]

The *IRS1 variant* increases the risk for insulin resistance[109] [111] *and TCF7L2 variants* is involved with insulin secretion.[110] If you have any of these variants, being aware of the type of carbohydrate you eat can be very important on your road in helping you lose weight. In fact, our nutrition team at Canyon Ranch would strongly encourage anyone who may have any of these variants to use a continuous glucose monitor. With this device, as explained in chapter 3, you can see what carbs cause a spike in your glucose. With that information you can either eliminate those particular carbs or change your meal composition to see if that levels off their spike. Remember, unlike the Keto diet in which one eliminates most carbs, a person can be more selective about their carbs, or what they are combining them with, if you use a monitor.

As you can see, there are some real advantages to knowing your genetic makeup. With the rapidly advancing science of genetics, the future is bright as to how we will use this branch of medicine to help guide our specific lifestyle patterns. There are many companies out there that perform nutrigenomic testing, and it can be a struggle to try to determine which ones are more valid and well-researched than others. Beware of those nutrigenomic companies that are affiliated with a food supplement company. The reason they are doing the test is to promote their products. This is also the case, as previously stated, with gut microbiome testing.

The study of genetics is what we call "upstream medicine." What I mean is that upstream you may be putting certain objects into your stream (your body) and making the assumption that it's going to create a specific product downstream. However, there are a lot of factors that can change your stream before it reaches its endpoint. You can add products that might improve and enhance the quality of your stream, or you can add bad products that may negatively affect the content of your stream's end-product. So knowing what is going on upstream as far as your genetics can help guide you about what to put into, or not put into, your stream.

The bottom line is that not everyone that wants to lose weight needs a genetic test. It is simply a deeper understanding of how and why our bodies work. It can give us a better understanding of why we have certain obstacles in our path to lose weight. I think one of the most important things that we can take away from this chapter is that information about your genetics helps you to understand why you may be struggling with your weight and others around you aren't. They can eat a bowl of ice cream every night and it does not seem to affect them, whereas just the thought of your eating ice cream at night seems to add five pounds to your belly. Ultimately the better we understand ourselves the easier it may be to address the problems that may arise.

13

Taking Stock and Moving Forward

Hopefully this book has separated itself from the many one-size-fits-all approach to weight loss and gives a more personalized method to getting rid of those unwanted pounds. There are plenty of programs out there that help a person lose weight, but they don't give enough tools to help the person keep that weight off. Most importantly, despite helping people lose weight, many of these other programs do not improve our overall health.

Most of the contemporary weight loss programs have one simple formula to lose weight. I wish it were that easy. People rarely become overweight because they did one thing wrong. Therefore, how can we expect to change only one thing to lose weight? Because of this, the path to attaining a healthy weight is not always an easy one. It takes some effort to get up out of that nice comfy warm bed in the morning to go for a run or give up that cheesecake that has your name written all over it. The reality is that we need to work at maintaining good health and losing weight. That is not necessarily all bad. We humans seem to appreciate things like good health more when we put a little effort into achieving it. As much as I personally don't enjoy exercising, to me there is no better feeling on the planet than that euphoric high I experience when I finish my run or my bike ride. It is just the best. I had to work to achieve that feeling, but my body loves me for it.

Let's summarize what you should do as you proceed on your path to a healthy weight. The very first thing you must do is to determine if there is a medical cause for your weight gain. You really can't start on a weight loss program until you have performed this first step. Please do not jump over this step and miss a medical etiology for the weight gain. If you do not address an untreated medical cause for the weight gain, your ability to lose weight is going to be much more difficult and could place you at an increased health risk. Therefore, if you feel there is an underlying medical issue potentially affecting your weight gain, please discuss it with your health care provider. Further testing may be warranted to rule out those medical causes. It is important to note that not all of the medical problems causing weight gain are serious health issues. In fact, once they are recognized, many of the medical maladies can have simple fixes. Some examples are changing to a medication that does not increase a person's appetite or treating an under-functioning thyroid with a once-a-day thyroid replacement medication.

After medical causes for weight gain are ruled out or discovered and treated, the next step in the quest for an experience of healthy weight loss is to focus on ways to attain the ideal goal numbers discussed in chapter 2. Meeting the goal number for pounds to lose is often important in improving a person's health. However, there are many other goal numbers important to attain in order to be considered healthy. It's important to have healthy blood pressure and cholesterol readings. It's good to have excellent fasting blood-sugar readings and insulin levels. The more in line you can be with the numbers you set with your doctor's approval, the more likely it will be that you'll be in a healthier state after your weight loss. A summary of these goals for your ideal numbers are at the end of chapter 2.

Once you have your goal numbers in focus and a good game plan on how to accomplish them, it's time to look again at the latest approach to healthy weight. The essence of this new approach is the realization that an individual's metabolic response to food can be different from person to person. Our response is dependent on several variables that include such things as food composition and their age and genetics. How someone responds metabolically can affect weight gain or loss and so can a person's overall health. We are able to analyze our individual metabolic responses to food by taking advantage of some of the new tracking devices such as a continuous glucose monitor. By understanding individually what foods and conditions cause different metabolic responses to foods, adjustments can be made in our meals, exercise, and emotional states to improve the metabolic reactions. With a normalized metabolic response to foods, a person can lose weight, improve overall health, and decrease the risk for future disease.

After determining what foods would be best for you metabolically, the next step is to look at your daily meal schedule. As discussed earlier, it has been determined that when we eat is almost as important as what we eat when it comes to weight loss. This is because of many factors, but one of the most important factors is related to insulin sensitivity. As was elucidated in chapter 4, insulin sensitivity is not stagnant during the day. In general, it has been shown that we are most sensitive to insulin at noontime, and it wanes as the day progresses. By knowing this, we can determine the amount and type of food a person should during their daily meals. Finally, in relation to mealtimes, it has been shown in many studies that it is generally best not to skip breakfast when trying to lose weight.

We show in this book that many aspects of our emotional health can affect our weight and overall health. Examples of this are seen in studies of people who are afflicted by emotional states of depression and anxiety. Both of these mental states have been associated with abnormal eating patterns. One of the most common of these patterns is excessive "emotional eating." Stress, depression, and anxiety often lead to this condition, and the result might be eating a whole box of cookies or a ½ gallon of ice cream at one sitting. If this is becoming a pattern, the underlining pathologic emotional state obviously should be addressed. We also learned that we need to be much more aware and mindful when we eat. This is a significant factor in weight gain that is often overlooked. We must be aware of the potential effects of bringing that bag of chips to the couch when we are watching TV or working on the computer. If we mindlessly eat, instead of mindfully eating, that whole bag of chips is gobbled up before we know it. We don't have to run to our favorite psychologist when this happens. The first step to deal with emotional eating and curb our mindless eating, is being aware that it is happening. If you are able recognize these abnormal eating patterns but are unable to stop yourself from continuing this abnormal pattern, it then may be time to seek out professional guidance.

Every year science learns more and more about the many intricacies of how our bodies function. With this knowledge, we have a better understanding today of the multitude of internal and external factors that can affect our weight and overall health. Scientists have discovered that the simplistic one-dimensional approach used for many years to get rid of those extra pounds—to just eat less and exercise more—is rarely the easy answer to losing weight. This is especially true for those who struggle with weight loss. As I've said, one of the newest areas of science utilized to help people lose weight is genetics. Knowledge of genetic factors gives insights as to why one person struggles with their weight and others don't. Genetics can be used to help guide a person in their food selections. Some individuals, for example, may be able to metabolize carbs better than fats or vice versa. With genetic information, we might direct an individual to the type of exercise program that would be better for them. They may be better designed genetically to do more high intensity exercises rather than low intensity, long-duration type of exercise programs.

Processed foods are another area that is being extensively studied. When they were originally produced and advertised, everyone thought this would revolutionize how we eat. Well, in many ways it was revolutionary, but unfortunately not all revolutions are necessarily good. Many of these processed foods were placed in boxes laden with preservatives that gave them a long shelf life. As far as convenience, it was great. But sadly, processed foods are often found to be unhealthy, and in many instances they have been associated with weight gain.

The use of artificial sweeteners in this country has exploded, and now 41% of the adult population uses some form of it daily. As discussed in chapter 11, several negative physiologic changes can happen in the body when consuming these food substitutes. The majority of the physiologic effects can result in weight gain. The simple solution to this is to do your best to avoid artificial sweeteners.

Lastly, the big new horizon in weight loss is the microbiome. Every day we are learning more and more about this incredibly complex matrix of trillions of bacteria that affect almost all aspects of the body's physiology. It has been shown to affect a person's mood, the absorption of fats and nutrients, the making of certain vitamins, the production of inflammation in the body, and a multitude of other functions, many of which we have yet to discover. The more we understand the microbiome, the better we are at manipulating it through personalized diets and possibly instituting specific pre- and probiotics to our daily intake.

I want to end this book as I started it. If you are trying to lose weight, your first goal is to improve your health. This will be accomplished by first treating any underlying medical issues and then systematically addressing the other topics discussed in this book. Finally, to obtain and maintain a healthy weight, you must continue to work at it on a daily basis. One does not become healthy and then magically stay healthy. It takes ongoing effort. If you are able to continue your efforts to remain healthy, it will pay you back in dividends many times over in improved longevity and a better quality of life.

Canyon Ranch Recipes

Created by Stephanie Miezin, MS, RD, CSSD
Canyon Ranch Director of Nutrition

How We Perceive Losing Weight

Weight loss for many can seem like a dreadful journey—full of restrictions and a lack of satisfaction—and filled with anxiousness around "falling off the wagon" because common weight loss tactics are simply unsustainable. The image of "diet" foods seems to be particularly loathsome: half a grapefruit with black coffee for breakfast, a no-frills salad with low-calorie dressing for lunch, maybe a solitary rice cake for a snack, the stand-by plain chicken breast with steamed broccoli for dinner, and definitely no dessert.

Of course, that level of restriction and one unappetizing meal after another is hardly sustainable. When it comes to eating, the great news is that losing weight and keeping it off can (and should!) be achieved through delicious, enjoyable foods. This strategy actually better plays into our natural biology, allowing you to use biology to your advantage rather than trying to constantly fight it. Understanding a little more about two major biological factors at play puts you in better control of your food and shifts eating from a negative to a positive light.

Food Mentality

In 2011, psychology researchers from Yale University and Arizona State University conducted a fascinating study centered on milkshakes. Participants consumed a moderate calorie (380 calorie) milkshake followed by measurement of their ghrelin, a hormone that produces the sensation of hunger and motivates food consumption. When the participants were told that the milkshake was higher calorie and "indulgent," their ghrelin levels were significantly lower after consumption, in contrast to participants who were told that the same milkshake was lower calorie and "sensible." This introduces the idea that perception of food can influence how satisfied we are after eating: thinking food is "lighter or healthier" leads to decreased satiety, while thinking of food as "indulgent or bountiful" leads to better satiety after eating.[111]

Use this insight to your advantage. Think about how you can switch the perspective on a meal from one of restriction to one of indulgence or nourishment. That mental shift can lead to you to feeling more satisfied after eating, which makes healthful eating more sustainable. For example, let's think of a meal that contains moderate portions of lemony roasted chicken, olive oil sautéed peppers and spinach with garlic, and caramelized sweet potato wedges. In a restriction mindset, thoughts about this meal might focus on the fact that there's no cheese topping the vegetables, feeling like chicken is boring diet food, or feeling the portions are too small in comparison to what may have been consumed previously. A mindset about nourishment would instead focus on the rich, varied flavors and textures of the meal and gratitude for the benefit that this nutritionally balanced plate will provide the body. Some knowledge about the many nourishing nutrients of foods strengthens this strategy of honing a mindset of valuing nutrition.

Understanding Metabolism

The human body requires energy to live and thrive. The process of turning food into that essential energy is what we call metabolism. Dieting commonly neglects the reality that adequate energy is non-negotiable. Instead of falling into less-is-more mentality for weight loss, let's dig a little into how a few key food components can nourish us with essential energy and more.

Protein

Protein is found in fish, poultry, dairy, eggs, soy, beans, and more foods. Dietary protein is vital to support a strong, healthy body. Without enough protein, muscle mass can decline. Losing muscle is usually not a good idea as muscle supports a healthy metabolic rate, physical functionality, and plays a big role in achieving desired appearances for many people. Protein takes a while to be digested, meaning it slows down the digestion of other foods in a meal too, like carbs. This insight is foundational when building balanced meals and snacks for great health and good blood glucose control.

Carbohydrates

Carbohydrates are found in grains, beans, fruits, vegetables, and other sources. Carbohydrates are the preferred fuel source of the brain and body. Consuming too few carbs can lead to low energy, irritability, inability to focus, and decreased physical performance. Low to no carb diets often promise weight loss. Weight loss may result, but it's not because carbohydrates are inherently "fattening." It's because reducing carbohydrates is a way to decrease energy consumed, potentially leading to an energy deficit and therefore weight loss. Including carbohydrates can, and almost always should, be part of a sustainable and enjoyable diet that supports optimal health.

Fat

Fat is found in nuts, seeds, oils, avocado, oily fish, and other sources. Fats help absorb fat-soluble vitamins (A, D, E & K), support hormone production, and provide long-lasting energy among other essential functions. Just like carbohydrates, fats themselves do not make people fat. (Too much fat, or any energy source for that matter, is what can lead to weight gain.) Fats, like protein, take a while to be metabolized. This results in important satisfaction after eating, as well as modulation of blood glucose response.

Fiber

Fiber is found in plant foods such as fruits, whole grains, vegetables, beans, nuts, and other foods. While the body does not really rely on fiber for energy, it does need it for good gut health. Many types of fiber act as food for the microbiota, making it essential for supporting a strong and diverse gut microbial community. Similar to protein and fat, fiber can slow digestion and contribute to increased satisfaction after eating, and even to better blood glucose control.

* * *

So, what are the implications of these biological insights for your weight loss goals, and how do we start to translate this to real food choices? Given the body's basic requirements for day-to-day life, extreme dieting or removing whole macronutrients or food groups is not necessary and realistically not sustainable. It can also lead to a restriction mentality and never feeling satisfied.

Instead, healthy and sustainable weight loss should be achieved with enjoyable meals that feel indulgent. An attitude of indulgence, our feeling that we treat ourselves to desirable meals, can be built by learning simple techniques that develop flavor at each step of cooking, creating irresistible flavor combinations and a meal composition that makes you feel great after eating. This is exactly what the following recipes have been designed to do.

These recipes are bursting with fresh flavor and are streamlined for minimal work and cooking time. They are strategically composed to result in better blood glucose control after eating and support healthful body composition, and they never leave you feeling restricted. These recipes are abundant in great nutrition that can support weight loss goals while also nourishing essential, foundational health.

Example of a Week of Healthful, Indulgent Eating

	Day One	Day Two	Day Three
Breakfast	Cherry Almond Baked Oats (pg. 142)	Mediterranean Frittata (pg. 145)	Blueberry Peanut Butter Smoothie (pg. 144)
Lunch	Seasonal Panzanella Salad with Roasted Chicken (pg. 150)	Sandwich - whole wheat bread, turkey breast, avocado and tomato. Side of fresh fruit	Chilled Miso Edamame & Broccoli Noodles (pg. 165)
Snack	Hard-boiled egg, string cheese, fresh berries	Cinnamon Almond Butter Protein Dip with Fruit (pg. X)	Greek yogurt with diced pear, pecans and pumpkin pie spice
Dinner	Tapenade Halibut with Garlicky Spinach and Chickpeas (pg. 159)	Sesame Crusted Chicken & Veggie Stir Fry Bowl (pg. 162)	Savory Grilled Mushroom & Steak Fajitas (pg. 160)
Dessert	Dark Hot Chocolate (pg. 172)		Instant Cherry Frozen Yogurt (pg. 173)

Day Four	Day Five	Day Six	Day Seven
Southwest Scramble Bowl (pg. 148)	Apple Walnut Overnight Oats (pg. 147)	Nordic Breakfast Sandwich (pg. 146)	Vanilla Pumpkin Smoothie (pg. 143)
Ginger Garlic Shrimp & Veggie Kabobs with Wild Rice (pg. 157)	Seared pork tenderloin, lemony broiled asparagus, herbed quinoa pilaf	Pressed Greek Feta Chicken Wrap (pg. 152)	Lemon Grilled Salmon with Garden Tabbouleh (pg. 151)
Smoked Salmon Crispy Cracker Bites (pg. 169)	Edamame hummus with cut veggies	Greek yogurt with berries and mixed seeds	Margherita Pizza Toast (pg. 170)
Herbed Turkey Meatballs with Roasted Tomatoes and Spaghetti Squash (pg. 154)	Chipotle Lime Chicken & Root Veggie Sheet Pan Meal (pg. 156)	Smoky Turkey Bean Chili (pg. 164)	Roasted chicken, garlic sautéed broccoli, peppery baked sweet potato
	Peanut Butter Chocolate "Cookie Dough" (pg. 174)		

Breakfast

Cherry Almond Baked Oats

Vanilla Pumpkin Smoothie

Blueberry Peanut Butter Smoothie

Mediterranean Frittata

Nordic Breakfast Sandwich

Apple Walnut Overnight Oats

Southwest Scramble Bowl

Cherry Almond Baked Oats

Makes 4 servings

4 cups ultra-filtered low-fat milk

¼ cup almond butter

¼ cup almonds, chopped or slivered

2 cups frozen cherries

1 cup steel cut oats

2 tsp. vanilla extract

¼ tsp. coarse/kosher salt

¼ tsp. ground cinnamon

2 cups non-fat plain Greek or Icelandic yogurt

Preheat oven to 375°F.

Choose a baking dish or loaf pan that can hold at least 2 quarts of liquid. A 9″ x 5″ loaf pan works very well.

Whisk the almond butter with half of the milk in the baking pan/dish until mostly incorporated. Stir in the rest of the milk and the remaining ingredients.

Cover with foil and bake for 75–90 minutes, until the liquid has been absorbed.

Serve warm with ½ cup Greek yogurt to make a balanced breakfast. Extras can be stored in the fridge for a couple of days and easily reheated in the microwave. Add a little water to thin out oats as needed before microwaving.

Nutrition per serving:
400 calories, 48g carbs, 23g protein, 15g fat, 8g fiber, 141mg sodium

Notes: Non-dairy milk can be substituted for the ultra-filtered cow's milk, but protein content will decrease unless a high-protein non-dairy milk is chosen. Choose certified gluten free oats to be sure this recipe is free of gluten. The final flavors will be different, but peanut butter could be swapped in for almond butter, other nuts can be used in place of the almonds, and other frozen berries or fruit could be used instead of cherries.

Vanilla Pumpkin Smoothie

Makes 1 serving

1¼ cup low-fat milk
½ cup pure pumpkin puree
1 tbs. almond butter
¾ scoop of vanilla protein powder
¼ tsp. vanilla extract
⅛ tsp. ground cinnamon or pumpkin pie spice

Combine all ingredients in a blender and blend until smooth.
A handful of ice can be added if desired.

Nutrition per serving:
400 calories, 48g carbs, 23g protein, 15g fat, 8g fiber, 141mg sodium

Notes: Choose a protein powder that has no added sugar and provides about 20g protein per scoop. Ultra-filtered milk could be used in place of traditional milk to increase protein content of this smoothie. A non-dairy milk could also be used in place of the cow's milk, but protein content of this smoothie may then be lower.

Blueberry Peanut Butter Smoothie

Makes 1 serving

¾ cup low-fat milk

¾ cup frozen blueberries

½ cup non-fat plain Greek or Icelandic yogurt

2 tbs. natural peanut butter

2 tbs. peanut butter powder

Combine all ingredients in a blender and blend until smooth. A handful of ice can be added if desired.

Nutrition per serving:
477 calories, 47g carbohydrates, 32g protein, 18g fat, 7g fiber, 175mg sodium

Notes: Ultra-filtered milk could be used in place of traditional milk to increase protein content of this smoothie. A non-dairy milk could also be used in place of the cow's milk, but protein content of this smoothie may then be lower. Other berries like strawberry or a berry blend could be used in place of the blueberries.

Mediterranean Frittata

Makes 4 servings

8 eggs
½ cup cottage cheese
2 oz. feta, crumbled
1 bell pepper, finely diced
½ cup artichoke hearts, finely chopped
¼ red onion, finely diced
2 tbs. basil, finely chopped
½ tsp. onion powder
½ tsp. garlic powder
½ tsp. black pepper
⅓ tsp. kosher/flaky salt

Heat oven to 350F.

In a large bowl, whisk eggs until smooth. Mix in the remaining ingredients until evenly combined.

Spray a glass baking dish (2-quart volume) with pan spray. Add the egg mixture to the dish. Bake for 35–45 minutes, until a fork comes out clean in the middle.

Balance out this frittata with whole grain toast and a side of fruit for a satisfying, nourishing breakfast.

Nutrition per serving:
234 calories, 8g carbs, 30g protein, 14g fat, 2g fiber, 560mg sodium

Notes: Other vegetables can be used in this frittata as well, like broccoli, spinach, kale, leeks, or asparagus. This frittata makes excellent leftovers. Store covered in the fridge for up to 3 days after making. Heat a slice for about 1 minute in the microwave to reheat.

Nordic Breakfast Sandwich

Makes 1 serving

2 slices of 100% whole wheat bread
1 egg
Black pepper
2 oz. smoked salmon
2 tbs. reduced fat cream cheese
½ cup arugula or baby spinach or kale
1 slice tomato
Thinly sliced red onion

Toast bread until desired doneness.

Heat a small sauté pan on medium-low heat. When hot, spray with pan spray. Crack egg into the pan and season with black pepper as desired. Cook until the egg appears to be halfway cooked, then flip over. Cook another 10≠20 seconds for a runny yolk, and 30–40 seconds longer for a fully cooked yolk. Remove from the heat.

Layer the salmon on one piece of toast. Top with the egg, greens, tomato and red onion, and then the other slice of toast. Enjoy right away.

Nutrition:
469 calories, 48g carbs, 33g protein, 19g fat, 8g fiber, 395mg sodium

Notes: Gluten free bread can be used in place of the whole wheat bread. Try to find a whole grain gluten free bread to still get the beneficial additional protein and fiber from the whole grains. Vegan egg can be scrambled and used in place of the whole egg if desired.

Apple Walnut Overnight Oats

Makes 2 servings

1 cup non-fat ultra-filtered milk

2 tbs. almond butter

1 cup non-fat plain Greek or Icelandic yogurt

1 cup rolled oats

1 apple, grated

¼ cup walnuts, chopped

2 tsp. chia seeds

¼ tsp. cinnamon

¼ tsp. vanilla extract

Pinch of kosher/flaky salt

In a medium to large container, whisk together the milk, almond butter and yogurt until mostly smooth. Add the remaining ingredients and continue mixing until evenly combined.

Cover container and place in the fridge overnight.

In the morning, enjoy oats chilled or heat in the microwave.

Nutrition:
517 calories, 54g carbs, 31g protein, 23g fat, 11g fiber, 132mg sodium

Notes: Non-dairy milk can be substituted for the ultra-filtered cow's milk, but protein content will decrease unless a high-protein non-dairy milk is chosen. Choose certified gluten free oats to be sure this recipe is free of gluten. The final flavors will be different, but almond butter could be swapped in for peanut or other nut butter and other fruit can be used in place of the apple, such as grated pear, fine diced peach, or frozen berries.

Southwest Scramble Bowl

Makes 1 serving

1 cup black beans, reduced sodium
1 poblano pepper, small diced
¼ cup grape/cherry tomatoes, halved
2 garlic cloves, minced
⅛ tsp. cumin, ground
⅛ tsp. chipotle powder (optional)
⅛ tsp. black pepper
Pinch of kosher/flaky salt
2 eggs
2 tbs. queso fresco, crumbled
1 tbs. cilantro, chopped (optional)

Rinse and drain black beans well. Place in a shallow bowl and set aside.

Heat a sauté pan on medium heat. When hot, spray well with pan spray. Add the poblano pepper and sauté for 2 minutes, until it starts to soften. Add the tomatoes, garlic, cumin, chipotle if using, black pepper and a pinch of salt. Cook for another 1-2 minutes, until garlic is very fragrant and tender.

Push veggies to one side of the pan. Spray the open side of the pan with pan spray. Crack the eggs into the open side of the pan. Use a spoon or spatula to move eggs around, scrambling them as they cook. When eggs are half cooked through, mix veggies into the eggs and cook another few moments until eggs are just cooked through. Remove from the heat.

Microwave the black beans for 1–2 minutes, until heated throughout. Top black beans with the veggie scrambled eggs, queso fresco and cilantro if using.

Nutrition:
492 calories, 51g carbs, 34g protein, 17g fat, 12g fiber, 590mg sodium

Notes: If poblano pepper is not available, look for an Anaheim chile, or even a small green bell pepper for less heat. Adjust the amount of chipotle powder to your desired heat level. A few portions of this dish can be made ahead of time and reheated for a quick breakfast over the next few days.

Lunch/Dinner

Seasonal Panzanella Salad with Roasted Chicken

Lemon Grilled Salmon with Garden Tabbouleh

Pressed Greek Feta Chicken Wrap

Herbed Meatballs with Roasted Tomatoes & Spaghetti Squash

Chipotle Lime Chicken & Root Veggie Sheet Pan Meal

Ginger Garlic Shrimp & Veggie Kabobs with Wild Rice

Tapenade Halibut with Garlicky Spinach and Chickpeas

Savory Grilled Mushroom & Steak Fajitas

Sesame Crusted Chicken & Veggie Stir Fry Bowl

Smoky Turkey Bean Chili

Chilled Miso Edamame & Broccoli Noodles

Seasonal Panzanella Salad with Roasted Chicken

Makes 2 servings

Dressing:

2 tbs. red wine vinegar

2 tbs. extra virgin olive oil

2 tbs. water

1 tbs. Dijon mustard

⅛ tsp. kosher /flaky salt

¼ tsp. fresh ground black pepper

Bread cubes:

2 cups 100% whole wheat bread, cut into 1" cubes

Salad:

8 oz. rotisserie chicken, pulled into bite size pieces (without skin)

4 cups baby kale and/or spinach

1½ cups seasonal fruit, cut into bite size pieces (apple, berries, peach, cherries, apricot, pear)

2 scallions, thinly sliced

Combine dressing ingredients in a small bowl, whisking until evenly combined. Set aside

Lay out bread cubes on a sheet pan and toast in an oven set to 350°F, or in a toaster oven. Cook until cubes are evenly golden on the outside and crisp. Let cool to room temperature.

In a large bowl, combine the bread cubes, chicken, baby greens, cut fruit and scallion. Add the dressing and mix all together very well until evenly combined and dressed. Portion into 2 bowls.

Nutrition per serving:
508 calories, 52g carbs, 41g protein, 18g fat, 9g fiber, 688mg sodium

Notes: Gluten free bread can be used in place of the whole wheat bread. Try to find whole grain gluten free bread for more fiber and protein. Tofu could be used in place of the chicken to make this dish vegan. Balsamic, white balsamic or white wine vinegar could be used in place of the red wine vinegar if desired. This salad is best enjoyed right after making.

Lemon Grilled Salmon with Garden Tabbouleh

Makes 2 servings

Tabbouleh:

⅓ cup bulgur wheat

⅔ cup hot water

½ cup parsley, finely chopped

¼ cup mint, finely chopped

1 medium tomato,
    small diced

1 cup cucumber,
    small diced

1 cup red bell pepper,
    small diced

2 scallions, thinly sliced

1 tbs. extra virgin olive oil

2 tbs. fresh lemon juice

⅛ tsp. kosher/flaky salt

⅛ tsp. fresh ground black pepper

Salmon:

2 each 4 oz. salmon filets,
    without skin

½ tsp. lemon zest

1 tsp. extra virgin olive oil

⅛ tsp. kosher/flaky salt

⅛ tsp. fresh ground
    black pepper

1 lemon, cut in
    half crosswise

Place bulgur wheat in a heat-proof bowl. Pour hot water over the grains, cover and let sit to absorb the water completely, about 20 minutes. Remove cover and let cool to room temperature. Add the remaining tabbouleh ingredients and mix together very well, until evenly mixed and dressed. Set aside until the salmon is done.

Preheat a grill or grill pan on medium-high heat.

Mix together the lemon zest, olive oil, salt and pepper. Spread over salmon to season evenly.

Place salmon on the grill with the presentation side facing down. Spray cut side of lemons briefly with pan spray and place cut side down on the grill.

Let salmon cook for ~3 minutes, until dark sear marks have developed and the salmon lifts easily when moved with tongs or a spatula. Rotate

90° and cook for another 2 minutes. Flip and cook another 1–2 minutes, until just cooked through. (Thicker pieces of salmon will take more time to cook through than thinner pieces. Salmon can be cooked to medium doneness if desired) Remove salmon and lemon from the grill.

Serve salmon with grilled lemon and the tabbouleh.

Nutrition per serving:
413 calories, 34g carbs, 28g protein, 19g fat, 4g fiber, 305mg sodium

Notes: Chicken, tofu or a white fish could be swapped in for the salmon. This dish is best enjoyed freshly made but could also be chilled and enjoyed over the next 1–2 days.

Pressed Greek Feta Chicken Wrap

Makes 2 servings

Herbed feta spread:

¼ cup low-fat plain Greek yogurt

¼ cup crumbled feta cheese

2 tbs. fresh basil, finely chopped

1 tsp. fresh garlic, minced

¼ tsp. fresh ground black pepper

Wrap:

2 medium (about 8″) whole wheat tortillas

6 oz. grilled or roasted chicken, cut into thin strips

1 cup arugula

½ cup canned chickpeas, reduced sodium,
    rinsed and drained well

½ cup roasted red pepper, cut into thin strips

¼ cup red onion, thinly sliced

Make the herbed feta spread by mixing together the yogurt, feta, basil, garlic and black pepper until evenly combined.

Spread equal amounts of the mixture on each tortilla, leaving 1" without spread around the edges.

Place 3 oz. grilled chicken, ½ cup arugula, ¼ cup chickpeas, ¼ cup roasted red peppers, and ⅛ cup red onion in the middle of each tortilla. Wrap tightly.

Heat a skillet on medium heat. When hot, place the wraps fold side down in the dry pan. Lightly press down on the wraps with a spatula. Let cook until golden on the bottom, flip and repeat.

Remove from the pan and cut each wrap in half crosswise. Enjoy right away.

Nutrition per serving:
368 calories, 27g carbs, 38g protein, 13g fat, 5g fiber, 738mg sodium

Notes: Tuna, salmon, turkey, tempeh or tofu could be used in place of the chicken if desired. A gluten free wrap can be used in place of the whole wheat bread. Try to find whole grain gluten free wraps for more fiber and protein. Arugula could be swapped out for baby kale or spinach. White beans could be used in place of the chickpeas. Hummus could be used in place of the herbed feta spread.

Herbed Meatballs with Roasted Tomatoes and Spaghetti Squash

Makes 4 servings

Spaghetti squash:

1 medium spaghetti squash

¼ tsp. fresh ground black pepper

⅛ tsp. kosher/flaky salt

Meatballs:

1 egg

½ cup whole wheat breadcrumbs

¼ cup fresh parsley, minced

¼ cup fresh basil, minced

¼ cup parmesan cheese, grated

2 tbs. garlic, minced

1 tbs. balsamic vinegar

¼ tsp. fresh ground black pepper

⅛ tsp. kosher/flaky salt

1 lb. 90% lean ground turkey or chicken

8 oz. grape/cherry tomatoes

¼ cup parmesan cheese, grated

Heat oven to 400°F.

Cut squash in half lengthwise. Scoop out the seeds and membranes. Season the inside with the salt and pepper, and spray cut flesh with pan spray. Place cut side down on a sheet pan. Roast in the oven for 45–55 minutes. Squash is done when a fork can be stuck through the flesh and skin easily. Remove from the oven and set aside.

Switch oven to broil to prepare for cooking the meatballs.

In a large bowl, whisk the egg until smooth. Mix in the breadcrumbs, herbs, Parmesan, garlic, balsamic, salt and pepper until evenly combined. Add the ground turkey or chicken, mix until just combined.

Portion out the mixture by heaping tablespoon (about 1 oz. each), roll into tightly packed balls, and place on a sheet pan (lined with foil for easier clean up) sprayed with pan spray. Allow at least an inch of space between each to allow for even cooking.

Place tomatoes on the pan interspersed with the meatballs.

Place pan in the oven under the broiler and cook for ~10 minutes, until tomatoes and meatballs are very golden. Meatballs should reach an internal temperature of 165°F.

Use a fork to scrape the flesh of the spaghetti squash crosswise to release the 'noodle' strands. Portion half of each half per person. Top with the meatballs, roasted tomatoes and Parmesan.

Nutrition per serving:
369 calories, 32g carbs, 30g protein, 17g fat, 6g fiber, 399mg sodium

Notes: Ground beef could be used in place of the chicken or turkey. Use gluten free breadcrumbs in place of the whole wheat breadcrumbs to make this meal free of gluten. Omit the parmesan to make this meal dairy free, or instead use nutritional yeast. Make this dish slightly simpler by omitting the roasted tomatoes and instead serving it with jarred tomato sauce.

Chipotle Lime Chicken & Root Veggie Sheet Pan Meal

Makes 2 servings

Sauce:
2 tbs. extra virgin olive oil
1 tbs. fresh lime juice
1 tbs. garlic, minced
½ tsp. lime zest
½ tsp. chipotle powder
½ tsp. cumin, ground
¼ tsp. fresh ground black pepper
⅛ tsp. kosher/flaky salt

2 medium boneless skinless chicken thighs (about 5 oz. each)
2 cups carrots, cut into ¾″ cubes or pieces
2 cups sweet potato, cut into ¾″ cubes or pieces
2 cups beets, cut into ¾″ cubes or pieces
1 lime, cut in half crosswise
¼ cup cilantro, rough chopped (optional)

Heat oven to 400°F.

In a small bowl, whisk together the sauce ingredients until evenly combined.

Line a large sheet pan with foil. Place cut veggies on the sheet pan and pour over ¾ of the sauce. Mix up well to evenly coat. Spread out veggies in an even layer on the pan, ideally with a little room between each piece to allow for even cooking. Leave some space on the pan for the chicken thighs.

Trim excess fat from the chicken thighs. Place on the sheet pan where there is space and rub on the remaining sauce. Fold chicken thighs up like a fist to encourage even cooking. Spray the cut side of the limes with pan spray and place the cut side down on the pan.

Place the sheet pan in the oven and roast for 35–40 minutes. Remove pan from the oven when the veggies are tender throughout and chicken is cooked to an internal temperature of 165°F.

Serve each chicken thigh with half the roasted veggies and a roasted lime half. Top with the chopped cilantro if using.

Nutrition per serving:

493 calories, 49g carbs, 33g protein, 20g fat, 12g fiber, 438mg sodium

Notes: Tofu steaks cut from firm tofu 1" thick could be used in place of the chicken, but protein content would decrease overall in the dish. Chicken breast could be used in place of the thighs but will likely be drier after cooking.

Ginger Garlic Shrimp & Veggie Kabobs with Wild Rice

Makes 2 servings

Rice:

½ cup wild rice, raw

¼ cup cilantro, minced (optional)

Kabobs:

1 tbs. garlic, minced

1 tbs. ginger, minced

1 tbs. extra virgin olive oil

1 tsp. sesame oil

¼ tsp. fresh ground black pepper

⅛ tsp. kosher/flaky salt

8 oz. raw shrimp, peeled

1 large zucchini or summer squash, cut into ½" rounds or half moons

1 large bell pepper, cut into 1" pieces

Several wooden skewers

Lime wedges

Fill a shallow bowl or container with water and place the wooden skewers in to soak for at least 10 minutes.

Rinse the rice very well with water. Place the rice and 2 cups water in a saucepan. Bring to a boil over high heat. Once boiling, reduce heat to medium-low to maintain a gentle simmer and cover the pan. Cook for 45–55 minutes. Test a few grains of rice at around the 45-minute mark. It is done when just tender throughout. Remove from the heat and drain in a fine mesh strainer. Return rice to the pot and cover, keeping warm until ready to serve.

Preheat a grill or grill pan over medium-high heat.

In a large container, mix together the garlic, ginger, oils, black pepper and salt until evenly combined. Add the shrimp, squash and bell pepper. Toss to evenly season the shrimp and veggies.

Preheat a grill or grill pan on medium heat.

Layer the veggies and shrimp onto the skewers. Place on the grill or grill pan. Cook undisturbed for 2–3 minutes, until the skewer easily releases from the grill when moved. Flip over and cook another 1–2 minutes, just until shrimp are white throughout, or to an internal temperature of 145°F.

When ready to serve, mix the minced cilantro into the rice if using. Plate rice along with the skewers and lime wedges.

Nutrition per serving:
422 calories, 44g carbs, 33g protein, 13g fat, 5g fiber, 470mg sodium

Notes: Chicken, salmon, lean beef or pork, or tofu cut into 1" cubes could be used in place of the shrimp. Cooking time will likely be a little longer for any of those other proteins. Quinoa, brown rice or other whole grain could be used in place of the wild rice if desired.

Tapenade Halibut with Garlicky Spinach & Chickpeas

Makes 2 servings

Tapenade:
¼ cup Kalamata olives, pitted
¼ cup basil leaves, loosely packed
1 medium garlic clove, chopped
1 tbs. fresh lemon juice
¼ tsp. lemon zest
⅛ tsp. fresh ground black pepper

2 each 4 oz. halibut filets, skin removed

Spinach and chickpeas:
2 tsp. extra virgin olive oil
2 tsp. garlic, minced
8 oz. baby spinach (about 6 cups loosely packed)
⅛ tsp. fresh ground black pepper
15 oz. can chickpeas, reduced sodium, rinsed and drained

Lemon wedges

Preheat the oven to 375°F.

Place tapenade ingredients into a food processor and blend until a paste is formed, scraping down the sides of the container as needed.

Place halibut filets on a sheet pan lined with parchment paper. Spread the tapenade over the top of the halibut filets. Place it on a middle rack in the oven and cook for about 10 minutes, until fish is just cooked throughout to 145°F.

While the fish is cooking, prepare the spinach. Heat a large pan on medium heat. When hot, add the oil and garlic. Cook, stirring constantly for 30 seconds. Add the spinach, season with pepper, and mix around in the pan well to encourage even cooking. When the spinach is mostly wilted, add the chickpeas. Continue cooking for 1 more minute, until spinach is just completely wilted and chickpeas are heated through.

Serve the halibut filets with the spinach-chickpea sauté and lemon wedges.

Nutrition per serving:
411 calories, 45g carbs, 35g protein, 13g fat, 16g fiber, 729mg sodium

Notes: This is best made with Kalamata olives, but could also be made with Castelvetrano olives if desired. Other fish like salmon or cod could be used in place of the halibut. Cooking times may vary when using other fish. If a food processor is not available, make the tapenade by very finely chopping the ingredients together for a few minutes. Kale could be used in place of the spinach. White beans could be used in place of the chickpeas. This dish is best enjoyed right after preparing.

Savory Grilled Mushroom & Steak Fajitas

Makes 2 servings

1½ tbs. soy sauce, reduced sodium

1 tbs. fresh lime juice

1 tbs. garlic, finely minced

½ tbs. extra virgin olive oil or avocado oil

½ tsp. fresh ground black pepper

½ tsp. cumin, ground

¼–⅛ tsp. cayenne or chipotle powder (optional)

6 oz. flank steak

2 portobello mushrooms, stem removed

1 bell pepper, any color, cut into quarters

4 green onions, roots trimmed

6 each 6" corn tortillas

½ medium avocado, cut into small cubes or thick slices

Fresh cilantro leaves

Lime wedges

Heat a grill or grill pan on medium-high heat.

In a shallow container, like a baking dish, mix together the soy sauce, lime juice, garlic, oil, black pepper, cumin, and cayenne or chipotle if using.

Add the steak, mushrooms, bell pepper and green onions. Mix with the sauce to evenly coat.

Place the steak on the preheated grill or grill pan. Let cook undisturbed for 2–3 minutes. Rotate the steak 90° and let cook for another 1–2 minutes. Flip and repeat. Cook steak to desired temperature, removing from the grill at 120°F for rare, 125°F for medium-rare, 130°F for medium, 140°F for medium-well, and 150°F for well done. Let rest while the veggies are cooked.

Place the mushrooms, peppers and green onion on the grill. Cook veggies until they have developed deep grill marks on the bottom, about 2–3 minutes. Repeat and cook until tender throughout, another 2–3 minutes.

Warm the tortillas on the grill if desired.

Thinly slice steak across the grain. Slice peppers and mushrooms into thin strips. Cut green onion into bite size pieces.

Serve steak and veggies with the tortillas and avocado, lime and cilantro to garnish.

Nutrition per serving:
445 calories, 47g carbs, 26g protein, 19g fat, 10g fiber, 504mg sodium

Notes: Chicken, beef or tofu can be used in place of the steak. Whole wheat tortillas could be used in place of the corn tortillas. Extra bell pepper can be used if omitting the mushroom. Leftovers can be chilled and reheated, but especially when using steak, these are best enjoyed right after preparing.

Sesame Crusted Chicken & Veggie Stir Fry Bowl

Makes 2 servings

½ cup quinoa

Chicken:

6 oz. chicken breast, thin slices about ½" thick

⅛ tsp. kosher/flaky salt

⅛ tsp. fresh ground black pepper

2 tbs. sesame seeds

1 tsp. extra virgin olive oil or avocado oil

1 tsp. sesame oil

Stir-fry:

½ tbs. extra virgin olive oil or avocado oil

1 tsp. sesame oil

1 red, orange or yellow bell pepper, cut into 1" pieces

½ cup onion, cut into ½" pieces

2 cups broccoli, cut into bite size florets

1 tbs. ginger, minced

1 tbs. garlic, minced

1 tbs. soy sauce, reduced sodium

1 tbs. balsamic vinegar

1 tbs. rice vinegar, unseasoned

Rinse the quinoa very well with water. Add to a saucepot with 1 cup of water. Turn heat to high to bring to a boil. Once boiling, turn heat down to medium-low to simmer gently and cover with a lid. Cook for 12–15 minutes, until quinoa grains no longer have white in the center and are tender when tested. Turn off heat and leave covered.

Prepare the chicken:

Season the chicken with salt and pepper. Sprinkle sesame seeds over chicken and lightly press to coat.

Heat a large sauté pan on medium heat. When hot, add the oils and swirl to coat the bottom of the pan. Place chicken in the pan with a little space between each piece. (Work in batches if pan is too small to fit all pieces of chicken at once) Let cook undisturbed for 2 minutes, until chicken is deep golden on the bottom and appears to be about halfway cooked. Flip and cook another 1–2 minutes, until the chicken is fully white throughout and reaches an internal temperature of 165°F. Remove chicken from the pan and reserve until ready to serve.

Prepare the veggies:

Use the same sauté pan to cook the veggies. Heat pan on medium-high heat. When very hot, add the oils and then peppers and onions. Sauté for 2–3 minutes, until peppers and onions start to brown and become more tender. Add the broccoli, ginger and garlic and cook for another 1≠2 minutes, until ginger and garlic are very fragrant.

Add the soy sauce, balsamic vinegar and rice vinegar. Mix well with veggies, allowing it to cook until the liquid has nearly evaporated. Remove from the heat.

Slice the chicken across the grain into thin strips. Place quinoa in bowls, top with the veggies and then the sliced chicken.

Nutrition per serving
482 calories, 47g carbs, 38g protein, 19g fat, 7g fiber, 439mg sodium

Notes: This recipe can easily be chilled and reheated for great meal prep or left-overs. Tofu could be used in place of the chicken, but sesame seeds likely will not stick as well. If using tofu, cut to about ¾" thick to focus on protein content. Cauliflower or asparagus could be used in place of the broccoli

Smoky Turkey Bean Chili

Makes 4 servings

1 tbs. extra virgin olive oil

1 cup onion, small diced

1 cup red bell pepper, small diced

2 tbs. garlic, minced

1 lb. ground turkey, 90-93% lean

1½ tbs. smoked paprika

1 tbs. chili powder

2 tsp. cumin, ground

2 tsp. oregano, dried

1 tsp. kosher/flaky salt

½ tsp. chili flakes

½ tsp. fresh ground black pepper

15 oz. can red kidney beans, reduced sodium, drained and rinsed

15 oz. can black beans, reduced sodium, drained and rinsed

15 oz. can crushed tomatoes

15 oz. can chicken stock, reduced sodium

½ cup cilantro, chopped

1 lime, quartered

Heat a large pot, such as a Dutch oven, over medium heat. When hot, add the oil, onion and bell pepper. Cook until the onion is translucent, a few minutes. Add the garlic and cook for another minute. Push veggies to one side of the pan.

Spray the open side of the pan with pan spray, then add the ground turkey. Let cook undisturbed for about 3 minutes, until dark golden on the bottom. Flip over and repeat. Use a spatula to break up the turkey into small pieces. Mix in the smoked paprika, chili powder, cumin, oregano, salt, chili flakes and black pepper.

Add the beans, crushed tomato and chicken stock. Bring to a rapid simmer, then decrease the heat to maintain a gentle simmer. Cook, stirring every few minutes for 45–60 minutes, until chili is thick and the flavors have fully developed.

Serve topped with cilantro and fresh squeezed lime.

Nutrition per serving:
433 calories, 44g carbs, 35g protein, 17g fat, 16g fiber, 623mg sodium

Notes: This dish is great for meal prep or leftovers and will keep in the fridge for up to 5–7 days. Ground chicken or beef could be used in place of the turkey if desired. Or, crumbled extra firm tofu could work well here too. If using tofu, this dish could be made completely vegan by using vegetable stock instead of chicken.

Chilled Miso Edamame & Broccoli Noodles

Makes 2 servings

Dressing:
1½ tbs. light or white miso paste
1½ tbs. rice vinegar, unseasoned
1 tbs. soy sauce, reduced sodium
1 tbs. sesame oil
2 green onions, thinly sliced

1½ cups shelled edamame
2 oz. whole-wheat spaghetti or linguini, dry
1 medium head of broccoli, cut into bite size florets

Bring a large pot filled ¾ full with water to a boil.

In a large bowl, mix together the dressing ingredients and add in the edamame. Set aside.

Drop the pasta into the boiling water. Cook, stirring occasionally, for 8–9 minutes. Once a tested noodle seems to need just about 1 more minute of cooking, add the broccoli to the pot. Stir well to encourage even cooking. Cook for just 1 minute, until broccoli is bright green.

Immediately remove from the heat and pour into a large colander set in the sink. Run cold water over the pasta and broccoli until completely chilled.

Add pasta and broccoli to the large bowl with the dressing and edamame. Mix everything together until evenly dressed and combined. Portion into bowls and enjoy.

Nutrition per serving:
408 calories, 50g carbs, 22g protein, 14g fat, 12g fiber, 528mg sodium

Notes: Increase protein in this dish by mixing in some roasted or grilled chicken or shrimp. Cauliflower or asparagus could be used in place of the broccoli. Gluten free noodles can be used in place of the whole-wheat noodles. Check the cooking instructions if using other noodles to see how the cooking time may need to be adjusted. This dish is great for meal prep, just make, chill and enjoy over the next few days.

Snacks

Cinnamon Almond Protein Dip with Fruit

Lemony Smoked Salmon Crispy Cracker Bites

Margherita Pizza Toast

Cinnamon Almond Protein Dip with Fruit

Makes 2 servings

¾ cup plain non-fat Greek or Icelandic yogurt

3 tbs. smooth almond butter

2 tsp. vanilla extract

½ tsp. cinnamon, ground

2 pieces of fruit, such as apple or pear, sliced into wedges

In a medium bowl, mix together the yogurt, almond butter, vanilla and cinnamon until evenly combined. Enjoy with the slices of fruit.

Nutrition per serving:
285 calories, 34g carbs, 16g protein, 14g fat, 7g fiber, 40mg sodium

Notes: Peanut or other nut or seed butter could be used in place of the almond butter. Non-dairy yogurt could be used, but protein content will likely be much lower. This is a great recipe to make a few portions of, store in the fridge, and enjoy for an easy snack over the next few days.

Lemony Smoked Salmon Crispy Cracker Bites

Makes 1 serving

2 tbs. part-skim ricotta cheese
½ tsp. fresh lemon juice
¼ tsp. lemon zest
⅛ tsp. fresh ground black pepper
1½ oz. smoked salmon
6 whole grain crackers
6 slices cucumber, about ¼" thick
1 tbs. fresh chives or green onion, thinly sliced (optional)

In a small bowl mix together the ricotta, lemon juice and zest, and black pepper.

Spread the lemony ricotta onto the crackers. Top each with a slice of cucumber and a piece of smoked salmon. Top with the chives or green onion if using. Enjoy right away.

Nutrition per serving:
261 calories, 23g carbs, 17g protein, 12g fat, 3g fiber, 192mg sodium

Notes: Make this dairy free by using a vegan ricotta or fine ground tofu. Other smoked fish like trout could be used in place of the salmon.

Margherita Pizza Toast

Makes 1 serving

1 slice 100% whole wheat bread
3 tbs. marinara sauce
1 oz. fresh mozzarella cheese
2 basil leaves, torn into small pieces

Heat a toaster oven to 350°F, or heat a broiler on medium.

Spread the marinara on the bread. Tear mozzarella into small shreds and arrange evenly on top of the sauce.

Place toast on a sheet pan if needed, and then into the toaster or under the broiler.

Cook for 3–5 minutes, until the bread is crisp, and the cheese is very melty.

Remove from the oven and top with the basil. Enjoy right away.

Nutrition per serving:
194 calories, 25g carbs, 11g protein, 7g fat, 5g fiber, 255mg sodium

Notes: Gluten free bread can be used in place of the whole wheat bread. Try to find whole grain gluten free bread for more fiber and protein. Slightly increase protein and decrease fat with reduced fat string cheese in place of the mozzarella. Fresh chopped tomatoes could be used instead of marinara sauce.

Desserts

Dark Hot Chocolate

Instant Cherry Frozen Yogurt

Peanut Butter Chocolate "Cookie Dough"

Dark Hot Chocolate

Makes 1 serving

¾ cup ultra-filtered non-fat milk

½ oz. dark chocolate (about 70% cocoa), broken into pieces or chunks/chips

1 tsp. dark Dutch processed cocoa powder

Heat milk in a microwave safe cup for 1 minute, until very hot.

Place chocolate and cocoa in a mug. Add a small splash of the hot milk into the mug, just enough to barely cover the chocolate. Let sit for 30 seconds.

Whisk very well so that the chocolate and cocoa powder are homogenous with the milk. Pour in the rest of the hot milk and mix well. Enjoy right away.

Nutrition per serving:
150 calories, 12g carbs, 11g protein, 7g fat, 2g fiber, 90mg sodium

Notes: Non-dairy milk can be used in place of the ultra-filtered milk, but this would most likely decrease the protein content of this beverage. Add a tiny bit each of cinnamon, cayenne and chipotle powders along with the cocoa powder to make this a Mexican inspired hot chocolate.

Instant Cherry Frozen Yogurt

Makes 2 servings

1½ cups frozen sweet cherries
½ cup low-fat plain Greek/Icelandic yogurt
1 tsp. vanilla extract

Place the cherries, yogurt and vanilla into a food processor. Blend, scraping down as needed, just until the mixture is smooth, about 1 minute. Don't blend too much longer, or else cherries will thaw too much. Enjoy right away.

Nutrition per serving:
132 calories, 19g carbs, 9g protein, 2g fat, 2g fiber, 28mg sodium

Notes: Non-fat or whole milk Greek yogurt could be used in place of the low-fat, but this will impact the nutritional content slightly.

Peanut Butter Chocolate "Cookie Dough"

Makes 10 servings

15.5 oz. can chickpeas, no salt added, rinsed and drained well

⅔ cup peanut butter powder

½ cup water

5 tbs. natural peanut butter

2 tbs. agave syrup or honey

⅛ tsp. kosher or flaky salt

Few dashes of cinnamon

5 tbs. dark chocolate chunks

Place the chickpeas, peanut butter powder, water, peanut butter, agave or honey, salt and cinnamon into a food processor. Blend, scraping down with a spatula as needed, until very smooth.

Add the chocolate chips into the food processor. Pulse several times until chocolate has visibly broken down into smaller pieces.

Enjoy hummus as is, or use as a dip for unsalted crackers or fruit like strawberries.

Store covered in the fridge for up to 5 days.

Nutrition per serving:
190 calories, 20g carbs, 11g protein, 9g fat,6g fiber, 195mg sodium

Notes: Almond butter may be used in place of the peanut butter. White beans could be used in place of the chickpeas.

Endnotes

1. https://www.cdc.gov/obesity/data/prevalence-maps.html.

2. Loos RJ., et. al. "The Genetics of Adiposity." *Curr Opin Genet Dev.* 2018;50:86. Epub 2018 Mar 9.

3. Frayling, T.M., Timpson, N.J. "A Common Variant in the FTO Gene Is Associated with Body Mass Index and Predisposes to Childhood and Adult Obesity." *Science.* 2007;316(5826):889. Epub 2007 Apr 12.

4. Samuels, M.H., Ridgway, E.C. "Central Hypothyroidism." *Endocrinol Metab Clin North Am.* 1992;21(4):903. Division of Endocrinology, University of Texas Health Science Center, San Antoni.; Andrea Lania et al. "Central Hypothyroidism." *Pituitary.* 2008;11(2):181. Department of Medical Sciences, Fondazione Ospedale Maggiore Policlinico IRCCS, University of Milan, Milan, Italy.

5. Martin I. Surks, MD, Douglas S. Ross, MD. "Clinical Manifestations of Hypothyroidism." Oct 2020.

6. Reynolds, G.P., McGowan, O.O. "Mechanisms Underlying Metabolic Disturbances Associated with Psychosis and Antipsychotic Drug Treatment." *Journal Psychopharmacol* (2017) 31(11):1430–6. doi: 10.1177/0269881117722987.

7. T. van Strien, et. al. "Emotional Eating As a Mediator Between Depression and Weight Gain." *Appetite*, 2016.

8. J.M. Murphy, et. al. "Obesity and Weight Gain in Relation to Depression: Findings from the Stirling County Study," *International Journal of Obesity*, 2009 Mar; 33(3): 335-341.

9. Lucia Alonso-Pedrero, et. al. "Obesity Management/Etiology and Pathophysiology Effects of Antidepressant and Antipsychotic Use on Weight Gain: A Systematic Review." *Obesity Review.* Vol. 20, issue 12. Pages 1680–1690.

10. Zumin Shi, et. al. "SSRI Antidepressant Use Potentiates Weight Gain in the Context of Unhealthy." *BMJ Open.* 2017; 7(8): e016224. Published online 2017 Aug.

11. Victor Maereel, et al. Front. "Psychotropic Medication Effects on Obesity and the Metabolic Syndrome in People With Serious Mental Illness," *Endocrinol.,* 09 October 2020, Impact of.

12. Virginio Salvi, Claudio Mencacci, et. al. "H1-Histamine Receptor Affinity Predicts Weight Gain with Antidepressants." *European Neuropsychopharmacology.* Volume 26, Issue 10. October 2016, Pages 1673–1677.

13. Reynolds, G.P., McGowan, O.O. "Mechanisms Underlying Metabolic Disturbances Associated with Psychosis and Antipsychotic Drug Dreatment." *Journal Psychopharmacol* (2017) 31(11):1430–6. doi: 10.1177/0269881117722987.

14. Davey, K.J., et al. "Antipsychotics and the Gut Microbiome: Olanzapine-Induced Metabolic Dysfunction Is Attenuated by Antibiotic Administration in the Rat." *Transl Psychiatry.* 2013;3:e309.

15. Ratliff, Joseph C., et al. "Association of Prescription H1 Antihistamine Use With Obesity: Results From the National Health and Nutrition Examination Survey." Obesity, vol. 18, no. 12, 2010, pp. 2398–2400., doi:10.1038/oby.2010.176.; Jørgensen, E., A., Knigge, U., Warberg, J., Kjær, A.: "Histamine and the Regulation of Body Weight." Neuroendocrinology 2007;86:210-214. doi: 10.1159/00010834.

16. Apovian, C.M., Aronne, L.J., Bessesen, D.H., et al. "Pharmacological Management of Obesity: An Endocrine Society Clinical Practice Guideline." J Clin Endocrinol Metab 2015; 100:342.

17. Leon I. Igel, Rekha B. Kumar, Katherine H. Saunders, Louis J. Aronne, "Practical Use of Pharmacotherapy for Obesity." *Gastroenterology*, Volume 152, Issue 7, 2017, Pages 1765–1779.

18. Daniele Sola, et. al. "Sulfonylureas and Their Use in Clinical Practice. *Arch Med Sci.* 2015 Aug 12; 11(4): 840–848. Published online 2015 Aug 11. doi: 10.5114/aoms.2015.53304

19. https://www.cdc.gov/nchs/data/hus/2017/058.pdf.

20. Lovejoy, J.C., et. al. "Increased Visceral Fat and Decreased Energy Expenditure During the Menopausal Transition. *Int J Obes (Lond).* 2008 Jun; 32(6):949–58.

21. Angelica Lindén Hirschberg.et. al. "Sex Hormones, Appetite and Eating Behavior in Women." *Maturitas. Review,* Vol., 71, Issue 3, P248–256, March 01, 2012.

22. Qian Gao, and Tamas L. Horvath. "Cross-Talk Between Estrogen and Leptin Signaling in the Hypothalamus." *Amer. Journal of Physiology Endocrinology and Metabolism* 01, 2008.

23. Wirasak Fungfuang, et. al. "Effects of Estrogen on Food Intake, Serum Leptin Levels and Leptin mRNA Expression in Adipose Tissue of Female Rats." *Lab Anim Res.* 2013 Sep; 29(3): 168–173.

24. Mary Fran Sowers, et al. "Change in Adipocytokines and Ghrelin with Menopause," *Maturitas*. Volume 59, Issue 2, 20 Feb. 2008, Pages 149–157.

25. Lovejoy, J.C., et. al. "Increased Visceral Fat and Decreased Energy Expenditure During the Menopausal Transition." *Int J Obes (Lond)*. 2008 Jun; 32(6):949–58.

26. D. Pu, R. Tan, et. al. "Metabolic Syndrome in Menopause and Associated Factors: A Meta-Analysis." *Climacteric*. 2017 Dec;20(6):583-591. Epub 2017 Oct 24.; Sezcan Mumusoglu and Bulent Okn Yildiz. "Metabolic Syndrome During Menopause." *Curr Vasc Pharmacol*. 2019;17(6):595-

27. Tikhonoff, V, et al. "The Uncertain Effect of Menopause on Blood Pressure." *Journal of Human Hypertension*. 2019;33:421.

28. Rachel R. Markwald, et. al. Physiology. "Impact of Insufficient Sleep on Total Daily Energy Expenditure, Food Intake, and Weight Gain." *Proc Natl Acad Sci USA*. 2013 Apr 2; 110(14): 5695–5700. Published online 2013 Mar 11.

29. Rachel R. Markwald, et. al. Physiology. "Impact of Insufficient Sleep on Total Daily Energy Expenditure, Food Intake, and Weight Gain. *Proc Natl Acad Sci USA*. 2013 Apr 2; 110(14): 5695–5700. Published online 2013 Mar 11.

30. Rachel R. Markwald, et. al. Physiology. "Impact of Insufficient Sleep on Total Daily Energy Expenditure, Food Intake, and Weight Gain." *Proc Natl Acad Sci USA*. 2013 Apr 2; 110(14): 5695–5700. Published online 2013 Mar 11.

31. Catherine G. Baaptiste, et. al. "Insulin and Hyperandrogenism in Women with Polycystic Ovary Syndrome." *Journal Steroid Biochem Mol Biol*. 2010, Oct;122(1-3):42–52.
    doi: 10.1016/j.jsbmb.2009.12.010. Epub 2009 Dec 28.; Unluhizarci, K., et. al. "Role of Insulin and Insulin Resistance in Androgen Excess Disorders." *World Journal Diabetes*. 2021;12(5):616-629. doi:10.4239/wjd.v12.i5.616.

32. Cassis L.A., et. al. "Local Adipose Tissue Renin-Angiotensin System." *Curr Hypertens Rep*. 2008;10(2):93-98. doi:10.1007/s11906-008-0019-9.

33. Nam, S.Y., Choi, I.J., Ryu, K.H., et al. The Effect of Abdominal Visceral Fat, Circulating Inflammatory Cytokines, and Leptin Levels on Reflux Esophagitis."
    Journal Neurogastroenterol Motil. 2015;21(2):247-254. doi:10.5056/jnm14114.

34. Andre Tchernof, et. al. "Pathophysiology of Human Visceral Obesity: An Update." *Physiological Reviews*. 01 Jan 2013.

35. Hardy, O.T., et. al. "What Causes the Insulin Resistance Underlying Obesity?" *Curr Opin Endocrinol Diabetes Obes*. 2012;19(2):81–87.
    doi:10.1097MED.0b013e3283514e13.

36. Willinam C. Cushman, Paul K. Wheaton, et. al. "Sprint Trial Results." *Hypertension.* 9 Nov 2015.

37. Kones R. et. al. "The Jupiter Study, CRP Screening, and Aggressive Statin Therapy-Implications for the Primary Prevention of Cardiovascular Disease." *Therapeutic Advances in Cardiovascular Disease.* August 2009:309-315.

38. Marc P. Allard-Ratick, et. al. "HDL: Fact, Fiction, or Function? HDL Cholesterol and Cardiovascular Risk." *European Journal of Preventive Cardiology*, Volume 28, Issue 2, February 2021, Pages 166–173.; Rosenson, Robert S., et. al., "Dysfunctional HDL and Atherosclerotic Cardiovascular Disease." Nat Rev Cardiol. 2016 Jan; 13(1):48060. Published online 2015 Sept 1.

39. Marc P. Allard-Ratick, et. al. "HDL: Fact, Fiction, or Function? HDL Cholesterol and Cardiovascular Risk." *European Journal of Preventive Cardiology*, Volume 28, Issue 2, February 2021, Pages 166–173.

40. Heo, Moonseong, et. al. "Percentage of Body Fat Cutoffs by Sex, Age and Race-Ethnicity in the US Adult Pop." From NHANES 1999–2004, *The Amer. J. of Clin. Nutr.* Vol. 95, Issue 3, March 2012, Pg. 594–602.

41. Zeevi, David. "Deciphering Postprandial Glycemic Responses in Human Subjects." Diss. The Weizmann Institute of Science (Israel), 2017.

42. Berry, S.E., et al. "Human Postprandial Responses to Food and Potential for Precision Nutrition." *Nat Med* 26, 964–973 (2020).

43. Lopez-Minguez, J., et. al. "Timing of Breakfast, Lunch, and Dinner. Effects on Obesity and Metabolic Risk." *Nutrients.* 2019;11(11):2624. Published 2019 Nov 1.

44. Daniela Jakubowicz, et. al. "High Caloric Intake at Breakfast Vs. Dinner Differentially Influences Weight Loss of Overweight and Obese women." *Obesity.* 20 March 2013.

45. Garaulet, M., et. al. "Melatonin Effects on Glucose Metabolism: Time to Unlock the Controversy." *Trends Endocrinol Metab.* 2020;31(3):192-204.

46. Lopez-Minguez, J., et. al. "Timing of Breakfast, Lunch, and Dinner. Effects on Obesity and Metabolic Risk." *Nutrients.* 2019;11(11):2624. Published 2019 Nov 1.

47. Keiko Asao, et. al. "Leptin Level and Skipping Breakfast: The National Health and Nutrition Examination Survey III (NHANES III)." *Nutrients.* 2016 Mar; 8(3): 115. Published online 2016 Feb 25.

48. Keiko Asao, et. al. "Leptin Level and Skipping Breakfast: The National Health and Nutrition Examination Survey III (NHANES III)." *Nutrients.* 2016 Mar; 8(3): 115. Published online 2016 Feb 25.

49. Lopez-Minguez, J., et. al. "Timing of Breakfast, Lunch, and Dinner. Effects on Obesity and Metabolic Risk." *Nutrients.* 2019;11(11):2624. Published 2019 Nov 1.

50. Jess A. Gwin and Heather J. Leidy. "A Review of the Evidence Surrounding the Effects of Breakfast Consumption on Mechanisms of Weight Management." *Adv Nutr.* 2018 Nov; 9(6): 717–725.

51. Leidy, H.J., et. al. "A High-Protein Breakfast Prevents Body Fat Gain, Through Reductions in Daily Intake and Hunger, in 'Breakfast Skipping' Adolescents. *Obesity* (Silver Spring). 2015 Sep;23(9):1761-4. doi: 10.1002/oby.21185. Epub 2015 Aug 4. PMID: 26239831.

52. Jess A. Gwin and Heather J. Leidy. "A Review of the Evidence Surrounding the Effects of Breakfast Consumption on Mechanisms of Weight Management." *Adv Nutr.* 2018 Nov; 9(6): 717–725.

53. Holly R. Wyatt, et al. "Long-Term Weight Loss and Breakfast in Subjects in the National Weight Control Registry." *Obes Res.* 2002 Feb;10(2):78–82.

54. Nicholas A. Christakis, M.D., Ph.D., M.P.H. and James H. Fowler, Ph.D. "The Spread of Obesity in a Large Social Network Over 32 Years." *N Engl J Med* July 26, 2007. 2007; 357:370-379.

55. Thibault Fiolet, et. al. "Consumption of Ultra-Processed Foods and Cancer Risk: Results from NutriNet-Santé Prospective Cohort. *BMJ* 2018; 360: k322. Published online 2018 Feb 14.

56. Leonie, Elizabeth. Et. al. "Ultra-Processed Foods and Health Outcomes: A Narrative Review," *Nutrients.* 2020 Jul; 12(7): 1955.

57. Marie Beslay, et. al. Ultra-Processed Food Intake in Association with BMI Change and Risk of Overweight and Obesity: A prospective Analysis of the French NutriNet-Santé Cohort." *Plos Med* 2020 Aug; 17(8): e1003256. Published online 2020 Aug 27.

58. Trepanowski, J.F., et. al. "Effect of Alternate-Day Fasting on Weight Loss, Weight Maintenance, and Cardioprotection Among Metabolically Healthy Obese Adults: A Randomized Clinical Trial." *JAMA Intern Med.* 2017; 177(7):930.; Varady, K.A., et. al. "Alternate Day Fasting for Weight Loss in Normal Weight and Overweight Subjects: A Randomized Controlled Trial." *Nutr J.* 2013;12(1):146. Epub 2013 Nov 12.

59. Tiffany A. Dong, MD, et. al. "Intermittent Fasting: A Heart Healthy Dietary Pattern?" *Am J Med.* 2020 Aug; 133(8): 901–907.

60. Detlev Boisin. "New Insights Into the Mechanisms of the Ketogenic Diet." *Curr Opin Neurol.* 2017 Apr; 30(2): 187–192.

61. Rhonda Ting, et. al. "Ketogenic Diet for Weight Loss. *Can Fam Physician.* 2018 Dec; 64(12): 906.

62. Crosby, L., et al. "Ketogenic Diets and Chronic Disease: Weighing the Benefits Against the Risks." *Front Nutr.* 2021;8:702802. Published 2021 Jul 16.

63. Hall, K.D., et. al. Effect of a Plant-Based, Low-Fat Diet Versus an Animal-Based, Ketogenic Diet on Ad Libitum Energy Intake." *Nat Med. 2021* Feb; 27(2):344–35).

64. Hall, K.D., et. al. "Effect of a Plant-Based, Low-Fat Diet Versus an Animal-Based, Ketogenic Diet on Ad Libitum Energy Intake." *Nat Med. 2021* Feb; 27(2):344–35).

65. Hall, K.D., et. al. "Effect of a Plant-Based, Low-Fat Diet Versus an Animal-Based, Ketogenic Diet on Ad Libitum Energy Intake." *Nat Med. 2021* Feb; 27(2):344-35).

66. Perdomo, C.M., et. al. "Impact of Nutritional Changes on Nonalcoholic Fatty Liver Disease." *Nutrients.* 2019;11(3):677. Published 2019 Mar 21.

67. Rena R. Wing, Suzanne Phelan. "Long-Term Weight Loss Maintenance," *The American Journal of Clinical Nutrition*, Volume 82, Issue 1, July 2005, Pages 222S–225S.

68. Aileen M. Pidgeon. et. al. "The Moderating Effects of Mindfulness on Psychological Distress and Emotional Eating Behaviour." *Australian Psychologist*}, {2013},volume 48, pages 262–269.

69. Jean L. Kristeller, et. al. Dept. of Psychology Indiana State University. "An Exploratory Study of a Meditation-Based Intervention for Binge Eating Disorder." *Journal of Health Psychology.* (1999). Vol 4 (3). 357–363.

70. Lisa S. Talbot et. al. "Post-Traumatic Stress Disorder Is Associated With Emotional Eating." *Journal of Traumatic Stress.* Published: 25 July 2013.

71. Sinha, R. "Role of Addiction and Stress Neurobiology on Food Intake and Obesity." *Biol Psychol.* 2018;131:5-13.

72. Yau, Y.H., et. al. "Stress and Eating Behaviors." *Minerva Endocrinol.* 2013;38(3):255–267.

73. Francesco Bottaccioli, et. al. "Brief Training of Psychoneuroendocrinoimumology-Based Meditation," (PNEIMED) Reduces Stress Symptoms Ratings and Improves Control on Salivary Cortisol Secretion Under Basel and Stimulated Conditions," *Explore (NY)* 10:3(2014):170-9. Kaipainen, K., et. al. "Mindless Eating Challenge: Retention, Weight Outcomes, and Barriers for Changes in a Public Web-Based Healthy Eating and Weight Loss Program. *J. Med. Internet Res.* 2012 Dec 17;14(6).

74. Kaipainen, K., et. al. "Mindless Eating Challenge: Retention, Weight Outcomes, and Barriers for Changes in a Public Web-Based Healthy Eating and Weight Loss Program." *J. Med. Internet Res.* 2012 Dec 17;14(6).

75. Steven R. Hawks, EdD., MBA, et. al. (2003) "Emotional Eating and Spiritual Well-Being: A Possible Connection?" *American Journal of Health Education*, 34:1, 30–33.

76. Eric S. Kim, Koichiro Shiba, et. al. "Sense of Purpose in Life and Five Health Behaviors in Older Adults." *Preventive Medicine*, Volume 139, Oct. 2020.

77. Leigh Perreault, MD and Michael Rosenbaum, MD. "Obesity: Genetic Contribution and Pathophysiology." *UPTODATE.* Updated December 7, 2021.

78. Darryn Willoughby, et. al. "Body Composition Changes in Weight Loss: Strategies and Supplementation for Maintaining Lean Body Mass, a Brief Review." *Annals of Internal Medicine.* April 4, 2017.

79. R.D. Varkevisser, et. al. "Determinants of Weight Loss Maintenance: A Systematic Review. *Obesity Reviews.* 2019 Feb; 20(2): 171–211. Published online 2018 Oct 16.

80. Aronne L.J., et. al. Describing the Weight-Reduced State: Physiology, Behavior, and Interventions." *Obesity* (Silver Spring). 2021;29 Suppl 1:S9.

81. Rosenbaum M., et.al. "Models of Energy Homeostasis in Response to Maintenance of Reduced Body Weight. *Obesity (Silver Spring) 2016;* 24:1620. Rosenbaum, M., et.al. Long-Term Persistence of Adaptive Thermogenesis in Subjects Who Have Maintained a Reduced Body Weight." *Am J Clin Nutr* 2008; 88:906.

82. Valensi, P., et. al. "Autonomic Nervous System Activity Changes in Patients with Hypertension and Overweight: Role and Therapeutic Implications." *Cardiovasc Diabetol* 20, 170 (2021).

83. Ursell, L.K., et. al. "Defining the Human Microbiome. "*Nutr Rev.* 2012;70 Suppl 1 (Suppl 1):S38-S44.

84. Mathur R. Barlow. "Obesity and the Microbiome." *GM Expert Rev Gastroenterol Hepatol.* 2015;9(8):1087. Epub 2015 Jun 16.

85. Yumei Xiong, et. al. "Short-Chain Fatty Acids Stimulate Leptin Production in Adipocytes Through the G Protein-Coupled Receptor GPR41," *Proceedings from The National Academy of Science of USA (PNAS)* January 27, 2004 101 (4) 1045-1050.

86. Paulina Markowwiak, et. al. "Effects of Probiotics, Prebiotics, and Synbiotics on Human Health." *Nutrients* 2017 Sep; 9(9): 1021. Published online 2017 Sep 15.

87. Ronald D Hills, et. al. "Gut Microbiome: Profound Implications for Diet and Disease." *Nutrients*. 2019 Jul; 11(7): 1613. Published online 2019 Jul 16.

88. Zmora, Niv; Segal, Eran; Elinav, Eran. The Pros, Cons, and Many Unknowns of Probiotics." *Nature Medicine*. 2019/05/01. 716- 729. VL1.

89. Sivamaruthi, Bhagavathi Sundaram et al. "A Review on Role of Microbiome in Obesity and Antiobesity Properties of Probiotic Supplements." *BioMed research international* vol. 2019 3291367. 9 May. 2019.

90. Monteiro, Cinara R. A. V., et al. "In Vitro Antimicrobial Activity and Probiotic Potential of *Bifidobacterium* and *Lactobacillus* against Species of *Clostridium*." *Nutrients* vol. 11,2 448. 21 Feb. 2019.

91. Markowiak P, Śliżewska, K. "Effects of Probiotics, Prebiotics, and Synbiotics on Human Health." *Nutrients*. 2017;9(9):1021. Published 2017 Sep 15.

92. Jason M. Ridlon, et. al. "Bile Acids and the Gut Microbiome." *Curr Opin Gastroenterol*. 2014 May: 30(3): 332-338.

93. Yuan Tian. "The microbiome Modulating Activity of Bile Acids." *Gut Microbes,* Pages 979–996 | Received 25 Oct 2019, Accepted 13 Feb 2020, Published online: 05 Mar 20.

94. Markowiak, P., Śliżewska, K. "Effects of Probiotics, Prebiotics, and Synbiotics on Human Health." *Nutrients*. 2017;9(9):1021. Published 2017 Sep 15.

95. De Preter V., Hamer, H.M., Windey, K., Verbeke, K. "The Impact of Pre- and/ or Probiotics on Human Colonic Metabolism: Does It Affect Human Health?" *Mol. Nutr. Food Res.* 2011;55:46–57.

96. George Washington University Milken Institute School of Public Health. "Consumption of Low-Calorie Sweeteners Jumps by 200 Percent in US children." *ScienceDaily*, 10 January 2017.

97. Steven D. Stellman, et. al. "Artificial Sweetener Use and One-Year Weight Change Among Women," *Preventive Medicine*, Volume 15, Issue 2, 1986, Pages 195–202.

98. Guy Fagherazzi, et. al. "Consumption of Artificially and Sugar-Sweetened Beverages and Incident Type 2 Diabetes in the Etude Epidémiologique auprès des femmes de la Mutuelle Générale de l'Education Nationale–European Prospective Investigation into Cancer and Nutrition Cohort." *The American Journal of Clinical Nutrition*, Volume 97, Issue 3, March 2013, Pages 517–523.

99. Jotham Suez, et. al. "Non-Caloric Artificial Sweeteners and the Microbiome: Fndings and Challenges." *Gut Microbes*. 2015; 6(2): 149–155. Published online 2015 Apr 1.

100. Alsunni, A. A. "Effects of Artificial Sweetener Consumption on Glucose Homeostasis and Its Association with Type 2 Diabetes and Obesity." *Int J Gen Med.* 2020;13:775-785. Published 2020 Oct 6. doi:10.2147/IJGM.S274760.

101. Jotham Suez, et. al. "Non-Caloric Artificial Sweeteners and the Microbiome: Fndings and Challenges." *Gut Microbes.* 2015; 6(2): 149–155. Published online 2015 Apr 1.

102. Abo Elnaga. et. al. "Effect of Stevia Sweetener Consumption As Non-Caloric Sweetening on Body Weight Gain and Biochemical's Parameters in Overweight Female Rats." *Annals of Agricultural Sciences.* Volume 61, Issue 1, June 2016, Pages 155-163.

103. Ruiz-Ojeda, Francisco Javier, et al. "Effects of Sweeteners on the Gut Microbiota: A Review of Experimental Studies and Clinical Trials." *Advances in nutrition (Bethesda, Md.)* vol. 10, suppl 1 (2019): S31-S48.

104. https://www.sciencefocus.com/the-human-body/how-to-boost-your -microbiome/

105. Wehby, G.L., Domingue, B.W., Boardman, J.D. "Prevention, Use of Health Services, and Genes: Implications of Genetics for Policy Formation." J Policy Anal Manage. 2015 Summer;34(3):519–36.

106. Katherine A. Fawcett, et. al. "The Genetics of Obesity: *FTO* Leads the Way. *Trends Genet.* 2010 Jun; 26(6): 266–274.

107. Helgeland, Øyvind, et al. "The Chromosome 9p21 CVD- and T2D-Associated Regions in a Norwegian Population (The HUNT2 Survey)." *International Journal of Endocrinology* vol. 2015 (2015): 164652.

108. Smith, Caren E., et al. "Apolipoprotein A2 Polymorphism Interacts with Intakes of Dairy Foods to Influence Body Weight in 2 U.S. Populations." *The Journal of Nutrition* vol. 143,12 (2013): 1865-71.

109. Feng, Xiang, et al. "Insulin Receptor Substrate 1 (IRS1) Variants Confer Risk of Diabetes in the Boston Puerto Rican Health Study." *Asia Pacific Journal of Clinical Nutrition* vol. 22,1 (2013): 150–9. doi:10.6133/apjcn.2013.22.1.09.

110. Zhou, Yuedan, et al. "TCF7L2 is a Master Regulator of Insulin Production and Processing." *Human Molecular Genetics* vol. 23,24 (2014): 6419–31.

111. Crum, A. J., Corbin, W. R., Brownell, K. D., & Salovey, P. (2011). "Mind Over Milkshakes: Mindsets, Not Just Nutrients, Determine Ghrelin Response." *Health Psychology: Official Journal of the Division of Health Psychology, American Psychological Association,* 30(4), 424–431. https://doi.org/10.1037/a0023467.

Index

ABOUT THE AUTHORS

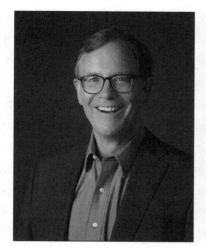 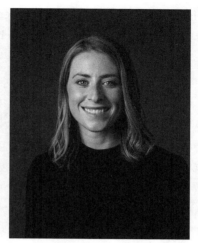

Stephen Brewer, MD, ABFM   Stephanie Miezin, MS, RD, CSSD

Dr. Stephen Brewer is the Medical Director of Canyon Ranch. He is a board-certified family physician who completed an associate fellowship in integrative medicine at the University of Arizona. He was trained and certified in Medical Acupuncture at UCLA and was trained and certified in guided imagery. He received his undergraduate degree from The Ohio State University, attended medical school at the Medical College of Ohio and completed his residency in family medicine at Riverside Methodist Hospital in Columbus, Ohio.

Dr. Brewer has been a physician in the medical field for 40 years. During that time he has worked in a wide variety of medical practice venues. He started his medical career as a country doctor in the Midwest. He then turned to teaching and became an assistant director of family medicine in a residency program teaching residents, interns, and medical students. He then went back into private practice in Cincinnati, Ohio and built one of the largest family practices in the greater Cincinnati metropolitan area. While he was in Cincinnati, in addition to his private practice, he became the first Medical Director of Integrative Medicine for TriHealth Hospital System. From there he moved to Tucson and became the Medical Director of Canyon Ranch where he has been since 2004. His areas of interest are Family Medicine, Preventive Medicine, Weight Loss, Integrative Medicine, Men's Health, and Complex Medical Syndromes.

Dr. Brewer is the author of the books *What Happened to Moderation?: A Common-Sense Approach to Improving Our Health and Treating Common Illnesses in an Age of Extremes; The Canyon Ranch Guide to Men's Health: A Doctor's Prescription for Male Wellness;* and coauthored *The Everest Principle: How to Achieve the Summit of Your Life.* He lectures on a regular basis to the guests at Canyon Ranch on topics that include "The Medical Approach to Weight Loss," "Men's Health," "Personalized Preventive Medicine," "Medically Undiagnosed Syndromes," "Reversible and Non-Reversible Dementia," and "Prevention of Heart Disease." He lectures nationally and internationally for various groups and medical institutions.

Stephanie Miezin is a Registered Dietitian and Certified Specialist in Sports Dietetics with experience in both dietetics and culinary arts. She has a bachelor's degree in culinary nutrition from Johnson & Wales University and a master's degree in medical dietetics from Ohio State University. Stephanie started out working in both the front and back of house of various restaurants and food service operations. She has worked for the USOPC fueling Team USA athletes by coordinating performance nutrition, recipes, and menus at Olympic and Pan American Games and at the Olympic & Paralympic Training Center in Colorado. She has also helped fuel athletes in the Tampa Bay Rays baseball organization, Ohio State University, and international soccer athletes. Stephanie is now the Director of Nutrition at Canyon Ranch.

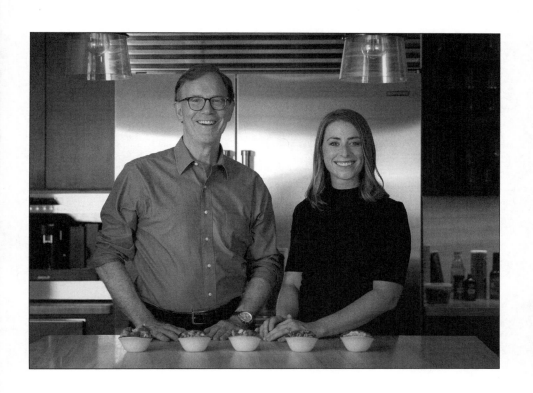